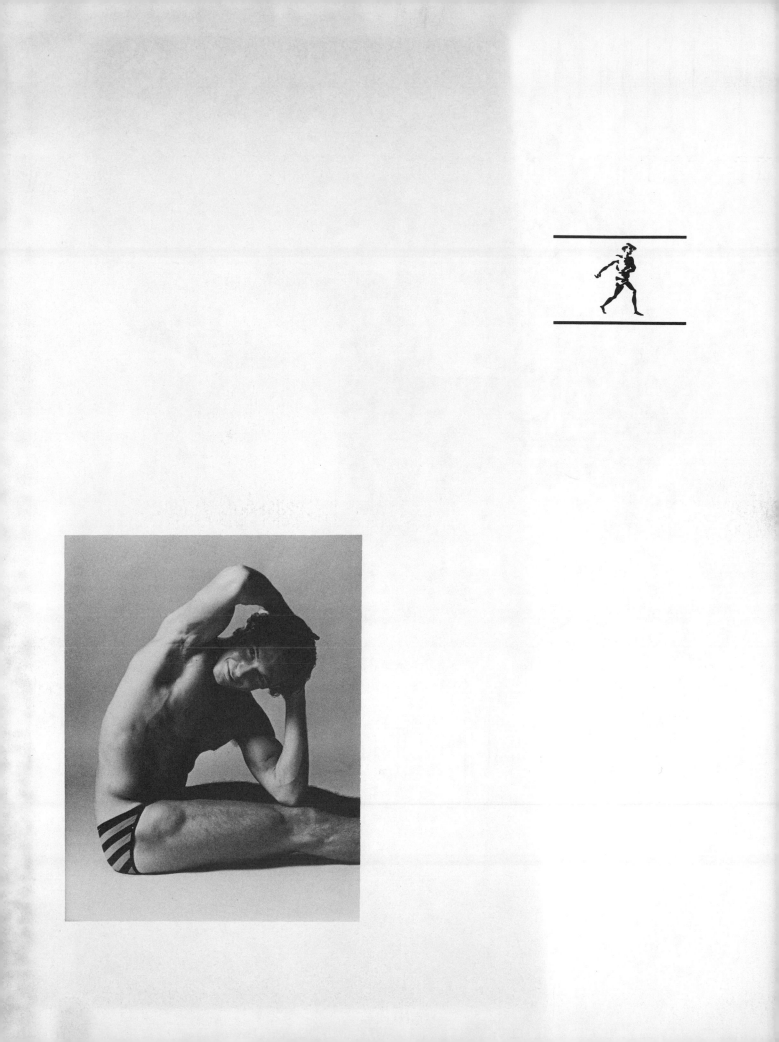

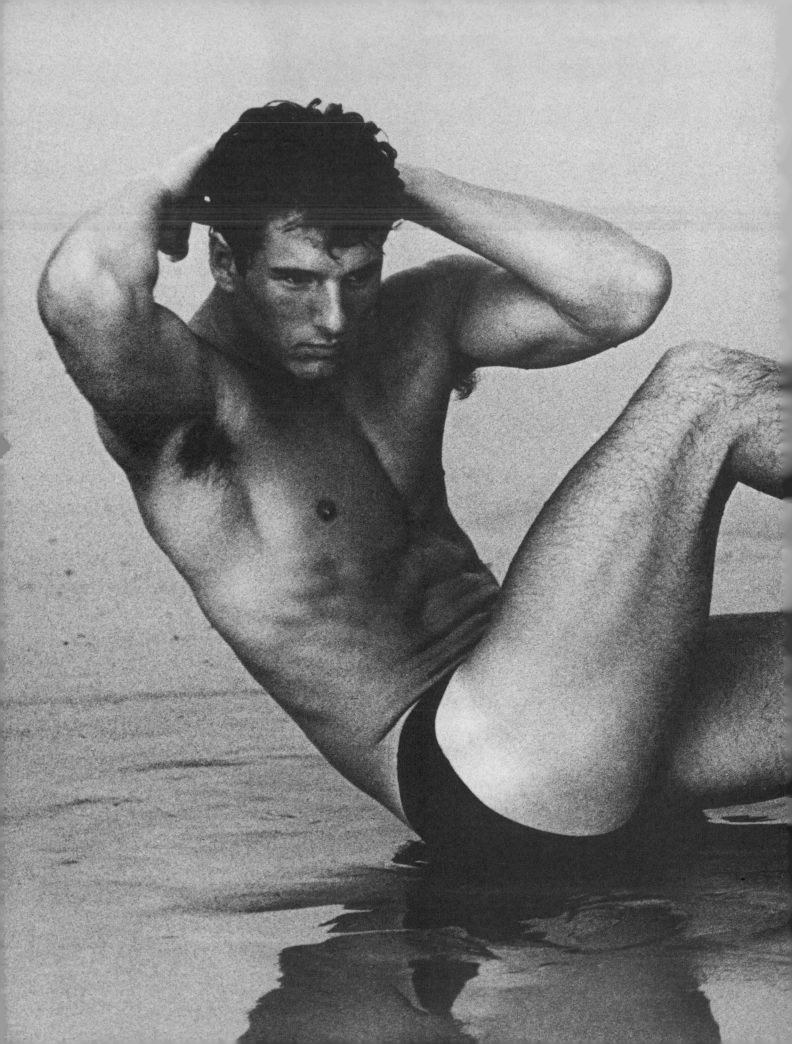

WORKING OUT

THE TOTAL SHAPE-UP GUIDE FOR MEN

BY

Charles Hix

Photographs by KEN HAAK

SIMON AND SCHUSTER

NEW YORK

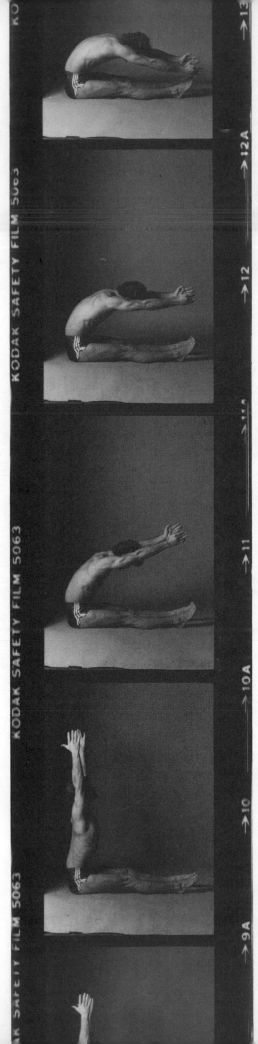

Published by Simon and Schuster
A Division of Gulf & Western Corporation
Simon & Schuster Building
Rockefeller Center
1230 Avenue of the Americas
New York, New York 10020
SIMON AND SCHUSTER and colophon are registered
trademarks of Simon & Schuster

Designed by Hix/Metz
Manufactured in the United States of America
10 9 8 7 6

Library of Congress Cataloging in Publication Data
Hix, Charles.
    Working out.
    1. Physical fitness for men. 2. Weight lifting.
3. Grooming for men.   I. Title.
GV481.H55 1983   613.7'044   82-19208
ISBN 0-671-45793-4

The author and the publisher of *Working Out* wish to ac-
knowledge the cooperation of The Athletic Complex, The
Body Center and the Chelsea Gym in providing locations
for photography; Donald Richardson for helping arrange
photographic locations; David Leong for supplying some
of the exercise fashions; and Marisa Stahovich for hair
styling. Special gratitude is expressed to all the modeling
agencies for their inestimable assistance.

To
KEN HAAK
for the intensity of his dedication
and for the power of his images;

TO
THE MODELS
David Allinson, Nic Andrews, Jim Bonner, Tom Brando, Craig Branham, Chris Byars, John Cunningham, Bob Dahlin, Dennis Decker, Jim Dugan, Barry Edward, Kem Edwards, Rick Edwards, Tom Ensign, John Ferris, Michael Flinn, Joey Gallinghouse, Terry Ganser, John Germaine, Bud Graves, Greg Gunsch, Jerry Gustin, Shawn Hammond, Dan Harvey, Tom Harvey, Mark Heller, Russell Henis, Jon Hensley, Kidane, Steve Kinsella, Jiles Kirkland, Stanley Lassak, Bob Lombardo, David Loring, Duke Lyskin, Peter Macci, Kevin McCoyd, Bill Meehan, Charles Melite, Kit Morris, Kevin Names, Mathew Nikitas, Matt Norklun, Michael Ordorica, George Patterson, Mark Peconi, Rick Popper, Steve Portello, Kevin Quinn, Ken Roberts, Jason Savas, Vincent Schenkel, Tony Silvers, Andrew Smith, David Spiewak, Dru Stevens, Randy Strong, Karl Szabo, Patrick Taylor and Doug Zane
for their unstinting help
and for their unwavering good humor;

TO
THE MASQUED BANDIT
for innumerable rewards
and for immeasurable riches.

CONTENTS

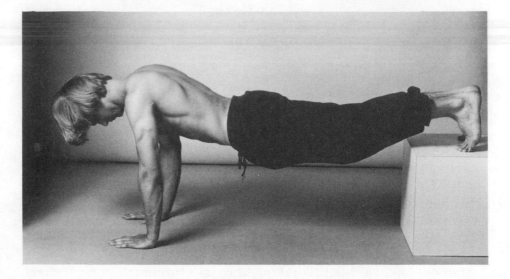

PART III

PRIDE & GROOM

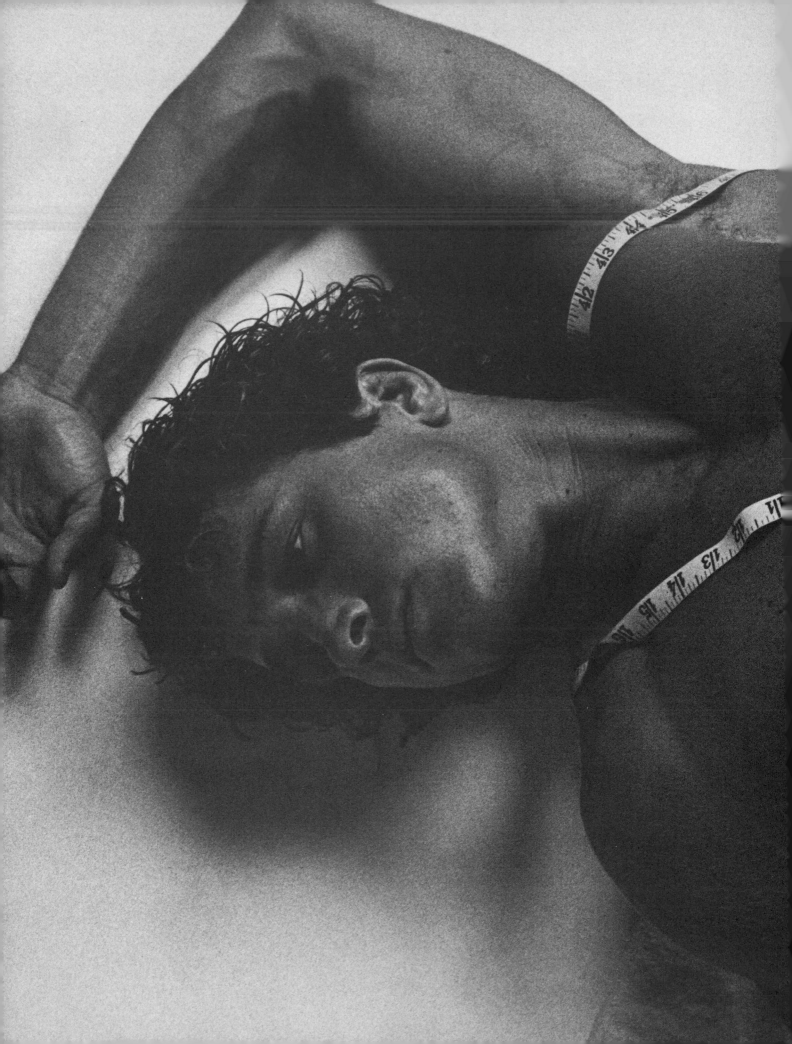

PART I
TAKING STOCK

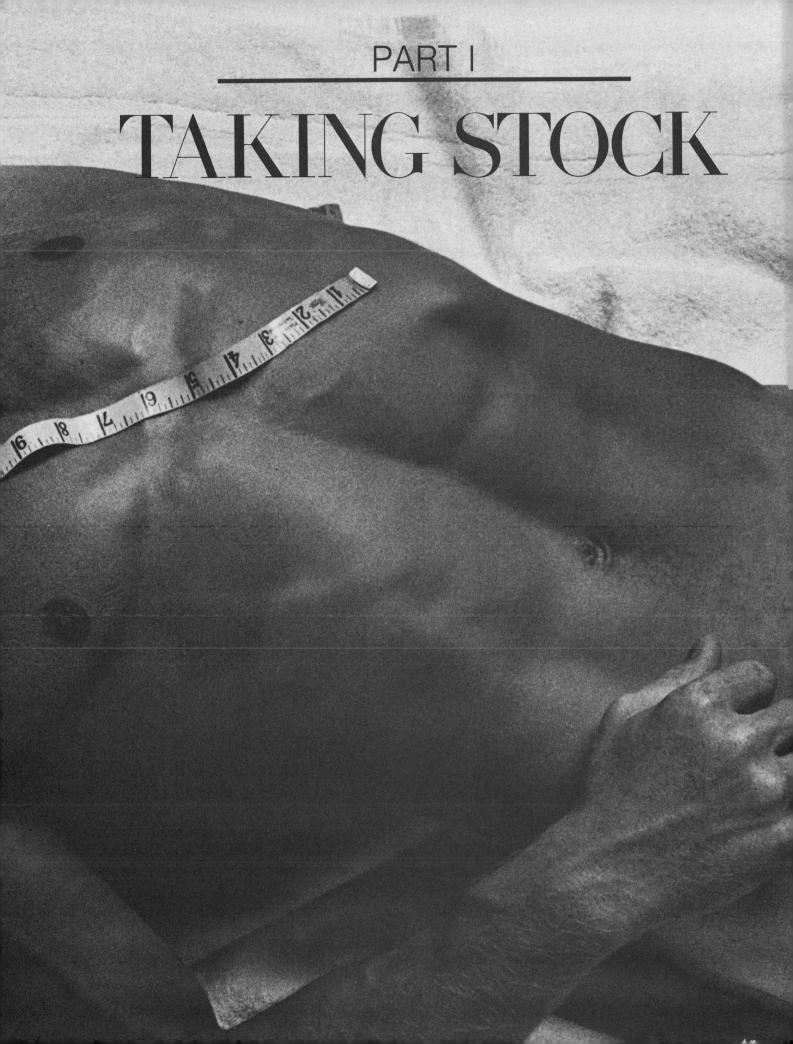

CHAPTER 1

STRIPPED AWAY

TRUE GRIT

To address your first question: Yes, you *can* shape up. The human body is a wondrous thing, and one of its wonders is the way it allows you to choose how you want to look.

To answer your next question. No, shaping up is *not* a piece of pie . . . but it gets easier as you go along.

If you can't accept the fact that working out is work, something that demands effort and grit, don't bother reading on.

Does that sound too stern? Sorry, but you may as well know where you stand. This book will not perform miracles. It can't infiltrate your psyche and fill you with determination you lack.

You say you really are committed to looking better? Prove it. Don't be a closet exerciser. Don't keep your decision to work out and shape up a secret. That's a sure signal that you're hedging your bet, keeping yourself covered in case you flub it. Don't even entertain the notion you can fail. You can't—

and won't—if you refuse to give up. Put your mouth where your mettle is: Tell everybody you know that you're off on a voyage of self-discovery, with working out your Baedecker.

That's no lie about self-discovery. You shouldn't try to turn yourself into somebody else, or somebody else's idea of what a great-looking male body encompasses. *Your* aim should always be to make the best of *you*, to discover your own potential and then to make the most of what you've got. To achieve that sense of euphoric accomplishment, you'll start out with cold facts on your side. Once you know the worst, you can be your best. Begin with brutal honesty.

FIRST IMPRESSIONS

Get acquainted with your own physique. By way of introduction, strip, preferably before a full-length mirror. Pretend you've never glimpsed any part of

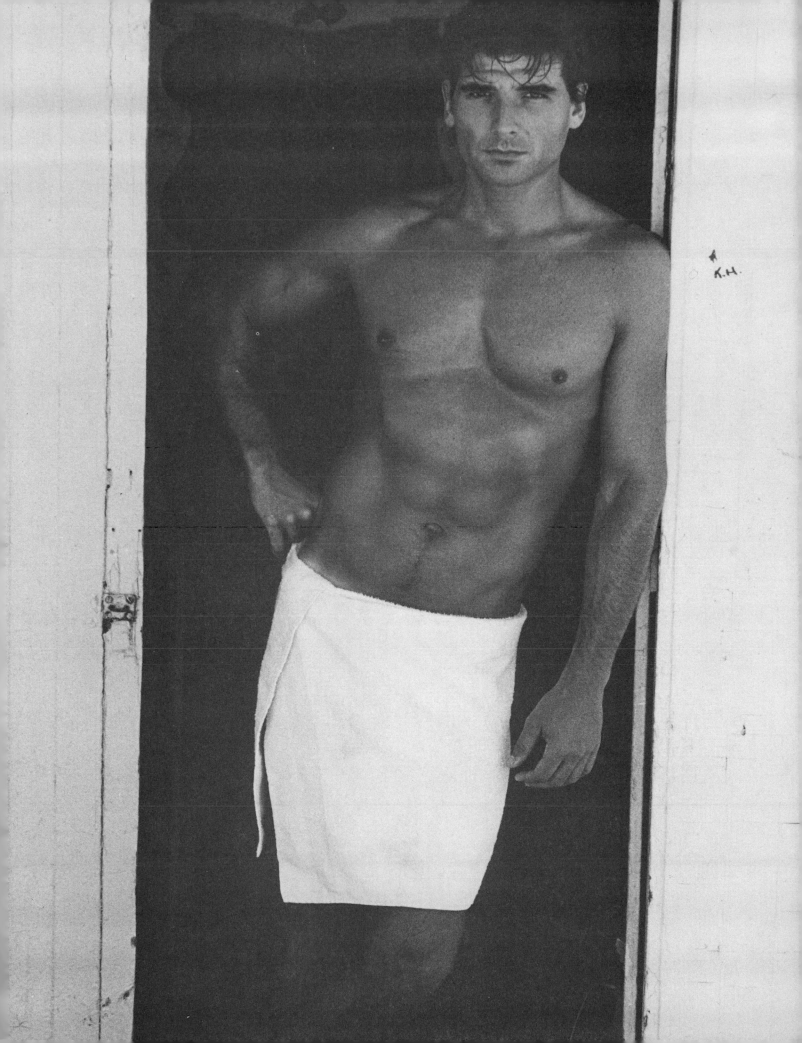

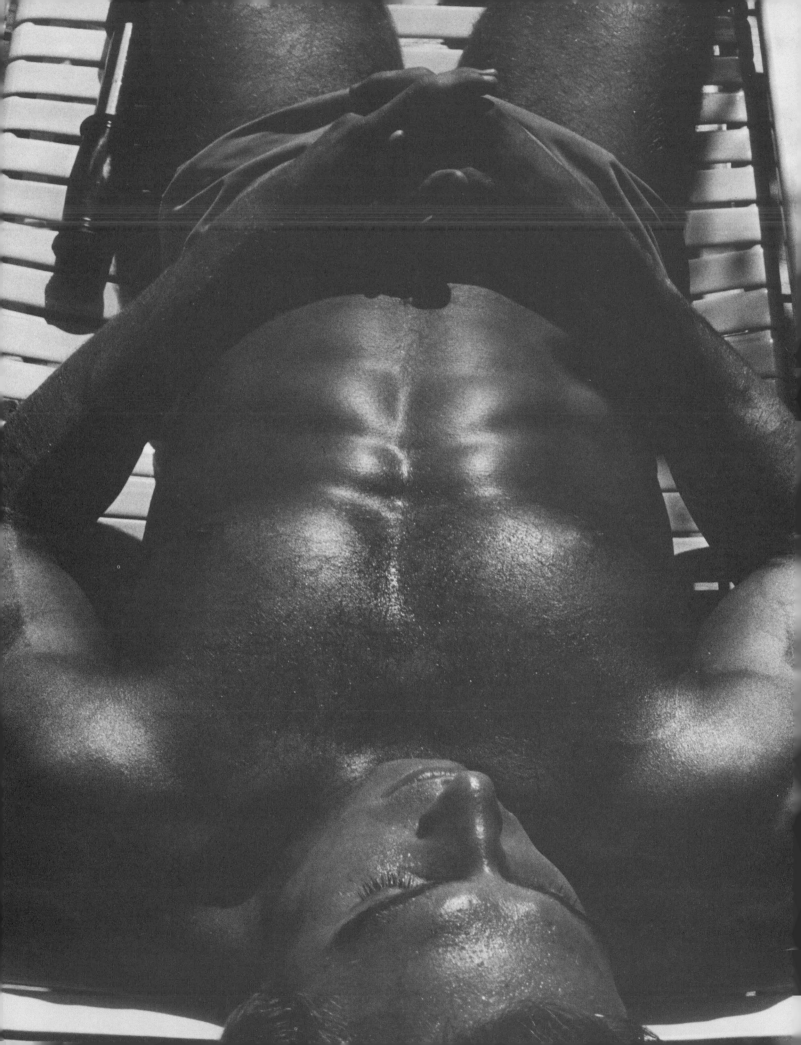

you before. Don't suck in your gut or adopt the stance of a private about to salute. Study your body as it really is, in repose, not as if you're posing in a Mr. Olympia competition.

Why bother going through this humbling routine? Because if you're like most men, you probably don't have a clear idea of what your body is really like.

Take inventory of yourself, making an honest assessment. Start out with your neck. Is it short and squat, long and swanlike, or somewhere in between? As you study yourself, be as objective as possible, noting each bulge, every crease. Move on to your shoulders. Are they broad, narrow, or simply there? Consider your chest. Does it swell or sink? What about your arms? waist? abdomen? legs? Isolate every part of you right down to your calves. For the moment, don't bother to score yourself on how great or not-so-great each part of your body is; just get a fix on how you're put together.

Now that you've examined this and that in detail, give yourself a sweeping head-to-toe glance. Turn to one side, then the other. Check out your rear view. How do you score yourself in toto after the quick scan?

That's the difficulty, isn't it? What should you compare yourself with when rating your physique? Certainly not Arnold Schwarzenegger's muscularity!

Although it sounds too simple, you should compare yourself with yourself.

Go back to the mirror. You don't need a chart listing ideal weights for specific heights to tell you if you're carrying too many or too few pounds. Your own eyes—and a good self-inflicted pinch at the waistline—will provide that answer. And your weight will further indicate whether you are—or aren't—living up to your own physical potential.

While examining yourself, keep in mind that your body is the product of both genetics (which you can't alter) and life-style (which you can). In fact, your life-style can have a profound effect on the visual aspects of genetic makeup: You may have been born with the genes of a Decathlon winner, but if your life-style has been that of Mr. Sedentary, your body will not appear Olympian. Conversely, genetically you may be predisposed to obesity, but

if you've always fought to control your appetite, you will probably be in far better shape than the man born with Decathlon-winning potential who has allowed himself to go to flab.

Here's how the foregoing observations affect you and your physique: You can't work yourself into *any* body configuration you choose, but every man has many more options than he realizes. Inbred limitations can't be totally overcome, but they can definitely be overshadowed: Even the most "average" male can sculpt a body of choice from his particular genetic clay.

However, don't think of your "inbred limitations." Instead, think about maximizing your inbred *potential.*

Back to the mirror.

Assuming you're in neither the best nor the worst of shape, what you see reflected in the mirror offers you a series of clues to your actual physical potential. Although you're unique, your body probably isn't. After all, some scientists insist that every human body can be categorized into one of three groups collectively called by the endearing term *somatotypes.* (*Somato-* refers to *body;* -*types,* in an uncharacteristic attempt at scientific and linguistic clarity, refers to *types.*) A body's *inborn inclination* to be muscled, to be rounded, or to be linear determines in which of the three slots it belongs. The "average" male body, according to the theory, is naturally inclined toward muscularity. It's what is commonly thought of as an athletically trim and toned physique, with more sinew than fat. (That may not be "average," but it's unquestionably the average man's goal.) A body's approximation of or deviation from this "average" physique decides the somatotype.

Needless to say, every individual is just that—an individual, with individual idiosyncrasies, including physical quirks. But underlying these variations, says the somatotype gospel, everybody and every body naturally veers toward *one* of the types more than the other two.

Take you, for instance. When you stood stripped before the mirror, which of these three adjectives most precisely described your reflection: Burly? Sinewy? Stringy? Don't argue. Choose *one* and one only.

BODY LANGUAGE

THE BURLY BODY

This is the type technically called an *endomorphic* body. The endomorph is born with a natural tendency toward a soft and round physique. Consequently, unless he works out to shape it otherwise, he probably has a relatively prominent abdomen. Left on its own, his muscular development doesn't seem pronounced, although he could be quite strong. His neck tends to be squat and his limbs shortish with fleshiness at the upper arms and thighs. He has a tendency to gain weight and to carry a large quantity of body fat. But when he

works out, he can look terrific, turning burliness to his advantage.

THE SINEWY BODY

This type, termed a *mesomorphic* body, is the "average" one with which the two others are compared. The appearance of musculature is the body's most pronounced feature. Shoulders and chest tend to be brawny, with highly developed arm and leg muscles and minimal body fat. Face it: Mesomorphs are the lucky ones genetically. If a man isn't born a mesomorph, he can never achieve true mesomorphy, although muscle can be built up through exercise. Of course, even a born mesomorph can go to pot. Mesomorphy, like the two other somato-

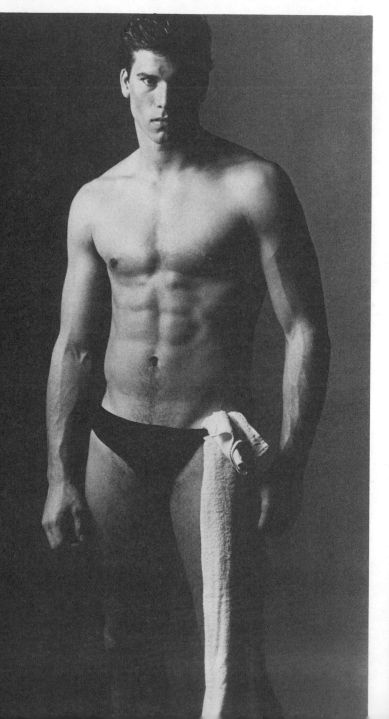 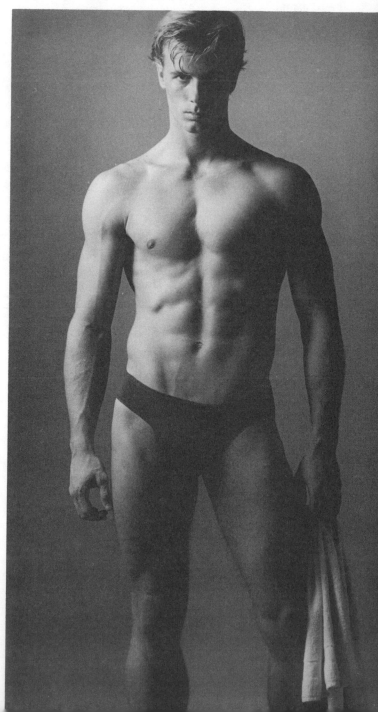

types, is an inherited inclination which can be obscured or enhanced by one's life-style.

THE STRINGY BODY

Typically lean, the *ectomorphic* body is naturally narrow and tends to be thin, with linear—as opposed to full-bodied—limbs. There is very little body fat. An ectomorph is usually tall, but not necessarily. And he needn't look like a Slim Jim. By working out, a fellow who otherwise might look stringy can look striking—just not striking in the same way that worked-out endomorphs or mesomorphs do.

Which somatotype do you most closely correspond to?

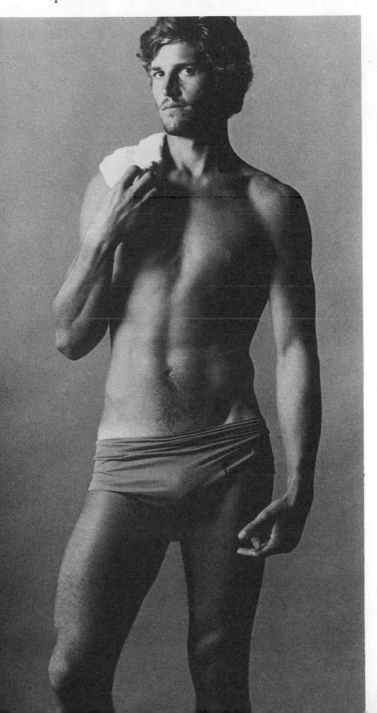

By recognizing your genetic somatotype, you're in a position to evaluate your body on its own terms rather than comparing yourself with some abstract notion of the Body Perfect . . . even though the "average" body of somatotypic theory isn't chopped liver.

Obviously, in the eyes of society, it's preferable to be born a mesomorph. But if you weren't, you weren't. It's pointless to rail against the injustices of biology. Yes, a mesomorph *does* have an inborn advantage. So what? Nonmesomorphs who work out can look better than true-blue mesomorphs who don't. Although you can't exchange your biological parents, you have a definite say in the visual consequences of their mating. You are not the pawn of fate.

Say you inherited a frame that swerves toward the burly. By jogging and dieting, by swimming and dieting, by jumping rope and dieting, by lifting weights and dieting, you *might* come across as somewhat of a mesomorph. But would it really be worth it?

Similarly, should your birthright prophesy a stringy adult body, by lifting weights and force-feeding yourself day in, day out, you *could* make yourself into a reasonable imitation of a mesomorph. But couldn't you find a more enjoyable—and profitable—way to fill your days?

Even if a sperm and ovum promised you a sinewy physique if you fertilized your potential, it's worth remembering that only one Mr. Olympia is crowned each year.

In short, there really is no one Body Perfect. You, and all other living males, were born with the capability to shape yourself either according to your own plan or according to happenstance. To repeat, you can't have *any* body in the world, but you can have a damn good one.

The wisest, fastest, and most efficient way to maximize your physique is to build upon your genetic legacy rather than going against your natural grain.

BURLY BODY. If your sojourn in front of the mirror informed you that you possess an endomorphic frame, recognize from the outset that to strive for a long and lean look is to court perpetual frustration.

One very satisfactory option is simply to follow a generalized fitness regimen to control your weight and to tone your body.

To make a larger physical statement by turning your natural propensity toward gaining weight to your advantage, you might seek a symmetrically squared, well-muscled body which needn't be slender to be attractive.

If your endomorphic tendencies are very pronounced, consider allowing yourself to carry more weight than customary while also carrying more muscle mass.

(Don't worry yet about how you're going to achieve the body proportions. That will come later. For now, simply try out the possibilities mentally.)

SINEWY BODY. If you were dealt this body type, your physical alternatives are more varied. For you, a generalized fitness routine will achieve a physique that appears gracefully strong.

To make a more specific impression, you might wish to emphasize your arm muscles . . . or your chest muscles . . . or whatever body areas you choose to make impressively presentable.

Similarly, you might decide to delineate your mesamorphy more strongly still by defining the musculature of your *entire* body.

(You could also go for broke and aim for a weight trainer's physique, but then you're off on a course outside the confines of this book.)

STRINGY BODY. Although your innate tendency is toward a long and lean frame, that's no reason you must look like a string bean. Simply by following a generalized fitness routine, you can easily aim for a physique with elongated, albeit understated, definition.

By taking advantage of the extra measure of endurance and stamina you possess by virtue of your body type, you could concentrate your efforts and dedication by working out certain particular muscles, maybe your neck and shoulders.

If you choose to work out your entire organism to its limit, it will be a long, hard climb, but with perseverance your body can achieve the proportions of a mythic lifeguard's.

OPTICAL ILLUSION

Here's the big surprise: The same exercises can be used by all body types to achieve their individual results. The harder you work out, the more pronounced—and visible—will be the results. *Your* optimum may not be someone else's, but you don't want to look like a clone anyway. When you build yourself up, you capitalize on your body's natural inclinations to accentuate your individuality. Unworked physiques fade into the anonymous masses.

The trick to a successful shaping-up system is no trick at all: By working out, you build up your body;

and by building up your body, you're dealing in optical illusion.

Think about it this way. When your body is flabby, it looks flabby. As you build up your whole body, your whole body looks—and is—less flabby. Moreover, as you continue working out, as your body takes on new dimensions, any physical shortcomings grow less and less evident. These shortcomings, which are becoming increasingly minor, still exist, but they are more than offset by your physical improvements. Your basic body type remains unaltered, but your body has become so enhanced that its drawbacks just aren't very apparent anymore. And that's optical illusion.

Very shortly you'll be introduced to a whole series of exercises to help you present your optimum physical self to your mirror and to the world. However, be patient for a little while longer.

The biggest mistake most men make in exercising is rushing into it without analyzing what they want, and understanding what they can expect. That's why most men quickly lose their resolve and why most of their efforts fail. Do yourself a favor. Learn some more before stampeding into the exercise section of this book. For the time being, read on.

CLOSE ENCOUNTER

You already know that your best bet in improving your body's appearance is to cash in on what nature passed your way rather than taking on the gargantuan task of trying to fit yourself into some body not your own. After all, whatever your raw material, there's a hell of a lot you can do with it.

On the other hand, even though your physical potential is great, how does the *current* status of your body truthfully rate? If there's a huge gap between the you whom you want to see and the you who's actually reflected in the mirror, then obviously you can't expect a transformation overnight. But even if you envision only minor realignment of your physique, you must take into account your present physical makeup, and that encompasses more than body dimensions.

If you've been very lax in the demands you've placed upon your organism, your endurance threshold may be moderate to minimal. Overtax yourself with a sudden ontake of rigorous activity and the consequences could be dire. So play it smart; be cautious.

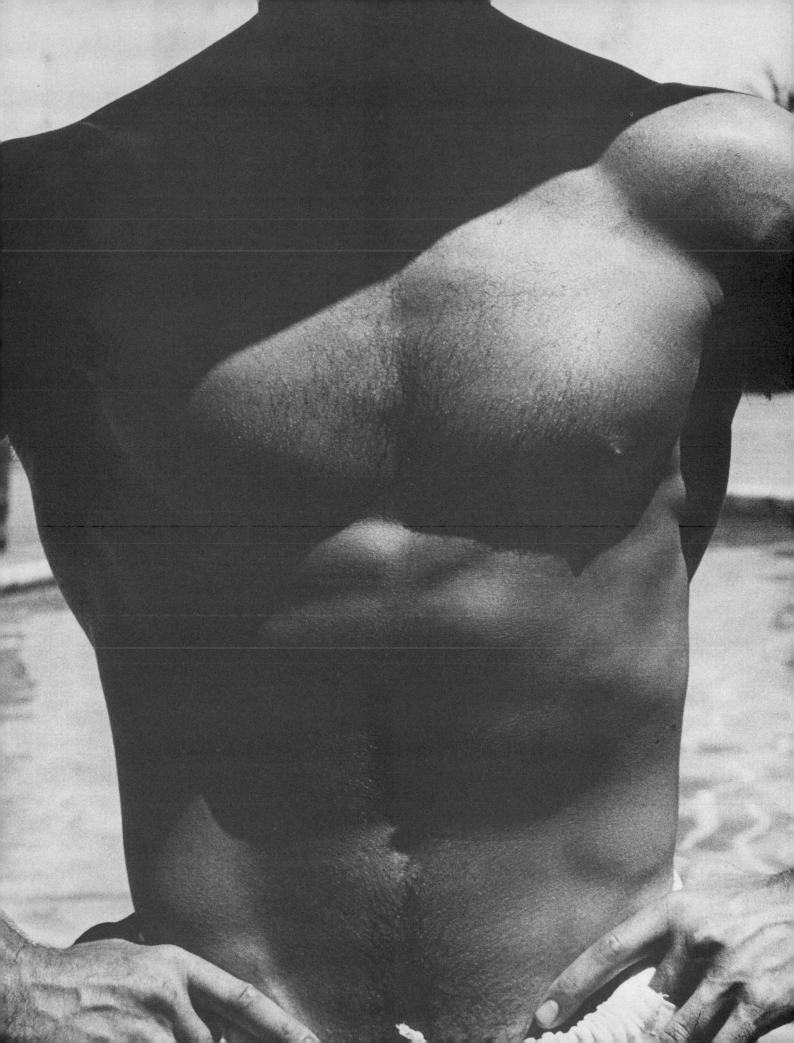

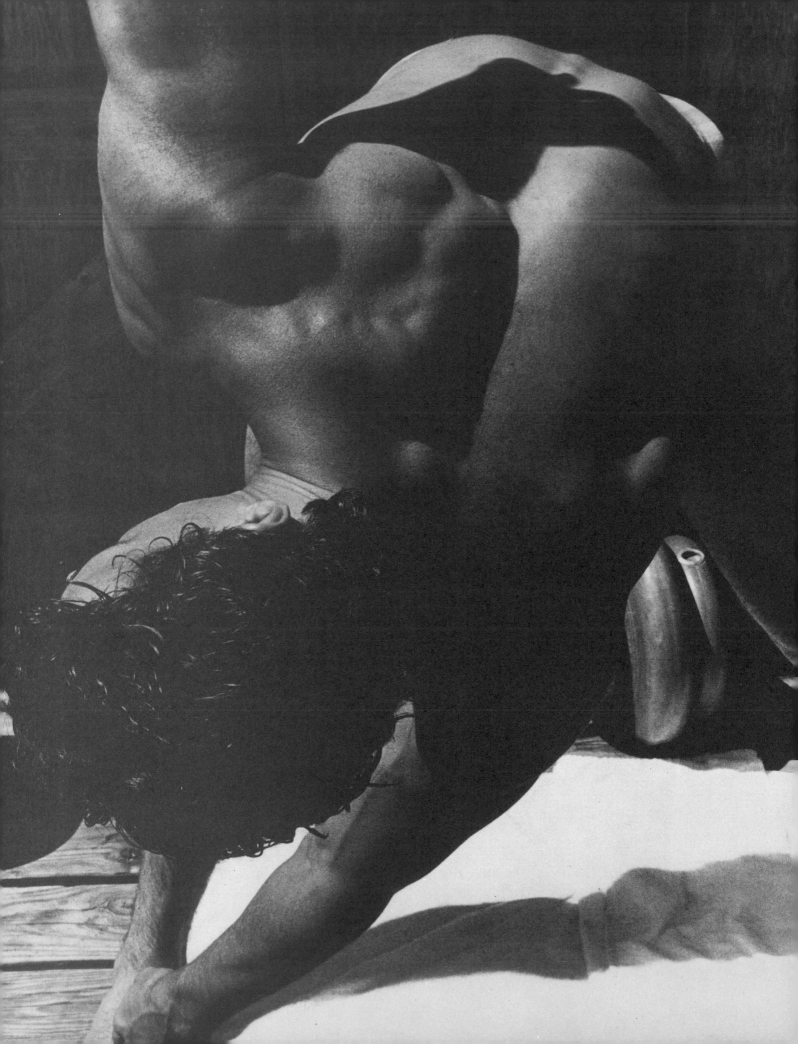

YOUR PULSE

Your pulse is the measurement of heartbeats. The more your ticker ticks in the space of a minute, the harder it's working, which means it's under greater stress. Whenever you stir yourself up from relaxed breathing to a pant or gasp, you're placing greater demands on your heart.

Taking your own pulse feels very alien at first; sometimes—initially, at least—it's difficult even to locate your pulse. Rest assured, if you had no pulse, you'd be in no position to measure it. But measuring it is extremely important, particularly if you plan to start working out after a prolonged period of physical inertia. Simply place the index and middle fingers of your right hand on the thumb side of your left wrist until you feel a slight throbbing or pulsating sensation. Using the second hand on a wristwatch, count the number of beats (starting the first one at zero) for fifteen seconds. Multiply that number by four and you have your resting pulse rate.

Don't procrastinate. Measure your pulse right now.

If your resting pulse is around 70 to 75, it's "normal," although a rate up to 90, while admittedly on the high side, could still be considered in the normal range. Above 90 is poor. On the other hand, a rate of 60 is excellent, a testimony to your physical fitness.

To illustrate why your pulse rate is so vital, consider this: The difference between a pulse rate of 60 and 90 is 30 beats per minute. In an hour, the difference is 1,800 beats. In a day, 43,200 beats. In a week, 302,400 beats. In a month, 1,209,600 beats. In a year, *14,515,200 beats.*

What this means is that a man whose pulse is 90 is calling upon his heart to beat fourteen and a half million more times in a year than a fellow with a pulse of 60 to do exactly the same thing—simply to exist!

What's more, when you're exercising, your heart beats faster than normal.

Fortunately, the human threshold is about 200 beats per minute without causing injury to the heart. But that would mean pushing yourself to the limit. Not smart. That's why almost anyone—particularly someone over thirty-five with no recent history of exercise—should have a stress electrocardiogram before embarking on any program of arduous activity. The conventional electrocardiogram, taken during rest, may not detect heart malfunctions that might be precipitated by exercise, but the stress electrocardiogram (taken under simulated exercise conditions) should.

This last point underscores why you must always be conscious of your pulsebeat, not only before initiating exercise but also during exercise. Although the goal of any legitimate working-out regimen must include lowering your pulse rate, thereby making your heart more efficient and resistant to injury, in order to reach that end you must first place additional stress on the heart—make it beat harder and faster, without overburdening it.

Although later you'll consider more variables, for the time being assume that the following formula will give you a fairly good indication of your *safe* maximum beating heart rate: Subtract your age from 200. (This allows for a safety margin, since generally the absolute maximum heart rate of the human body is 220.) If you're twenty, your safe maximum pulse is 180 (200 minus 20); if you're thirty, it's 170 (200 minus 30); forty, 160; et cetera. Your maximum beating heart rate is a limit you'll *never* purposely surpass. In fact, you'll choose to remain *under* that maximum. However, to train your heart for progressively more arduous exercise, for limited periods every day you will definitely push it past your resting pulse rate. (More specific information on how to use your heartbeat as a guide during various stages of exercise will be given in Chapter 8.) With time, you may actually succeed in

SMOKING

Is there any man alive who doesn't know smoking cigarettes has nothing to recommend it?

If you don't give a fig about the incompatibility of smoking and working out, skip this section. If you're interested in why they're incompatible, proceed.

Addictive nicotine, which in strong doses is lethal, stimulates the heart to beat more often, whereas a slowing of the pulse is one of the most desired ends of working out. But it isn't nicotine alone that causes the heartbeat of smokers to climb.

One of the gases released in the lungs by cigarette smoke is carbon monoxide (another killer in strong-enough concentration). It is so seductive to the hemoglobin in the blood that it combines more rapidly with it than oxygen does. Hemoglobin is supposed to carry oxygen through the body, but when useless carbon monoxide displaces some of that helpful oxygen, the oxygen content in the bloodstream is reduced. (Smoking also cuts down on the efficient intake of oxygen into the respiratory system in the first place.) The heart has to pump harder to get less oxygen than it wants, so it pumps harder still.

Not a pretty story, is it?

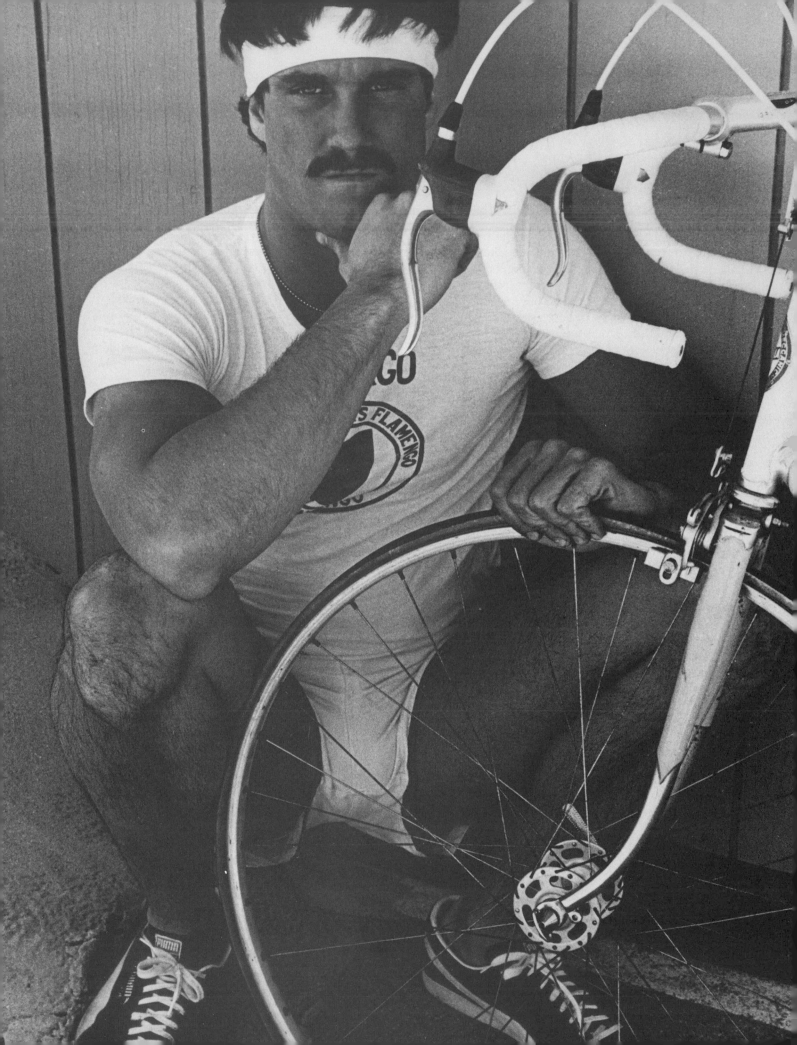

lowering your resting heartbeat, thereby enhancing your heart's efficiency and your overall fitness. Plus, you'll have a healthier-looking, better-toned body.

AEROBIC FITNESS

The word *aerobic* refers to oxygen. Aerobic fitness is a measure of your body's ability to utilize oxygen efficiently. Any activity that improves the performance and endurance of the heart and lungs (commonly called the cardiovascular system) will affect your heartbeat. (To be long-winded and correct, technically aerobic fitness depends upon the functioning of the cardiovascular-respiratory system. For ease—ease?—let's just call it the cardiovascular system.)

Improving aerobic fitness is the first requirement of working out. But, as just noted, your current aerobic fitness must dictate the speed with which you can safely and sanely proceed. If you feel bushed after climbing a ladder to replace a defunct light bulb overhead, or if your heart is pounding to beat the band after you lunge into an animated polka, you are not aerobically fit. Bad posture and pains in the back and legs often indicate that one's aerobic fitness isn't all it should be. Excessive weight is almost always a sign of unfitness.

FLEXIBILITY

Just as aerobic fitness protects the heart from injury, limber muscles protect the body from injury. The longer muscles go unused, the shorter and tauter they become; they quite literally shrink. In this reduced state, they can't stand up to even minimal trauma. A short sprint after a departing bus could be so shocking that several muscles could tear or be otherwise damaged. The lesions may be small enough that you'll not even know they're there—until the next morning, when they'll be so touchy you won't want to disturb them.

With appropriate exercise, even atrophied muscles stretch again. As they elongate, they become more elastic. Given a shock—another dash after that departing bus, for example—they are literally more able to bounce back into action without great hardship.

The more you ask of your muscles, the more limber they must be. Shoveling snow off a long, steep driveway with unstretched arms and back is no fun.

Any beneficial working-out routine must incorporate ways to increase muscle flexibility; but as with aerobic fitness, gently does it at first if the body isn't primed.

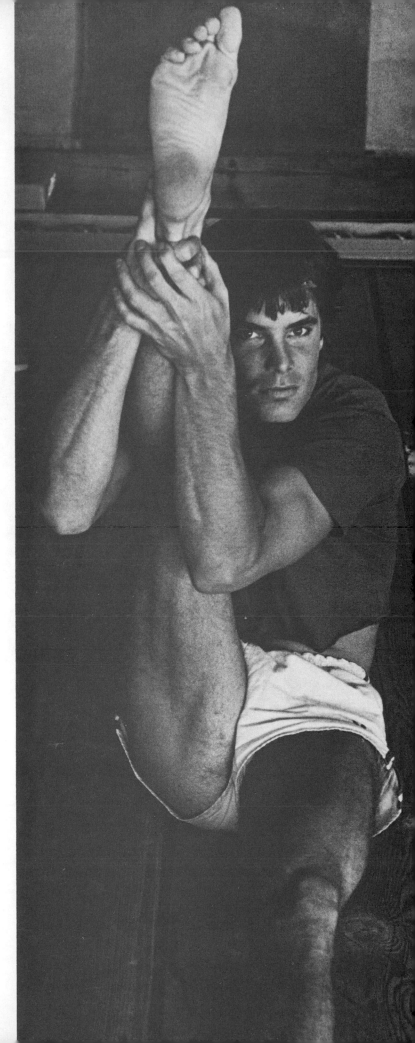

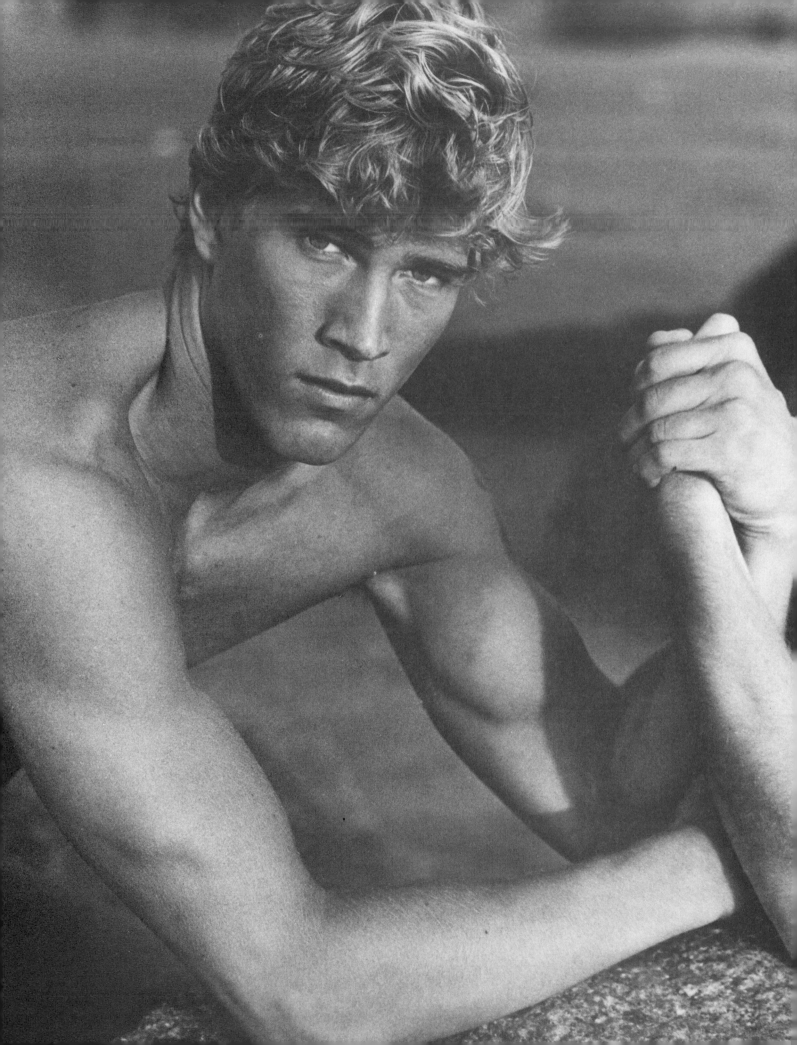

STRENGTH

Your cardiovascular system could be pumping away efficiently and your muscles might be flexible as all get-out, but your ability to heft an overpacked suitcase from the floor could be nil. While modern times seldom require astonishing deeds of brute strength, it never hurts to have muscle power in reserve. Also, the only way to build muscle mass is to strengthen your body simultaneously.

If you can't lift a heavy suitcase, you shouldn't contemplate pressing three hundred pounds in the immediate future. But only by forcing your body to exceed itself will you excel. Whenever you stop placing demands on your muscles, they get lazy. Think about what happens to long-term bedridden convalescents. Their muscles wither from disuse. To a lesser degree, the same phenomenon occurs with desk-ridden executives whose only long-term exercise is pushing a Dictaphone button.

Strength doesn't come from popping vitamins or swallowing eggs raw. It comes from work—muscle work.

ENDURANCE

Let's say you can lift that overpacked suitcase after all. It might not be a big deal to lift it, but is it a picnic lugging it for a mile?

Exertions of strength that take only a second or two won't work out the cardiovascular system, but they may place great strain on underdeveloped muscles. Anytime you call on your muscles to do more than they're accustomed to, and you make them perform that onerous task over a period of time to boot, you're asking for muscle endurance you may or may not have. If you're lacking muscle power to begin with, you certainly can't endure any strenuous labor for long. Similarly, if you think you have Samson's strength but you've allowed your cardiovascular fitness to deteriorate, despite those prizewinning pecs, you shouldn't charge into sustained strenuous labor either. (Actually, if you've gotten that badly out of shape, your pecs probably aren't all that prizewinning, unless you're a steroid freak.)

Your body works at its best only when you keep working it out. Muscle is as muscle does. This is an aphorism that works. To maximize yourself, you must maximize your strength. Combine strength with cardiovascular health and you get *real* endurance.

JOB APPRAISAL

Without specialized equipment found only in fitness laboratories, there's no surefire way to get more than a general fix on the various components of your present physical condition. Lots of do-it-yourself methods exist, though none of them is perfect. Among the most popular is The 12-Minute

AGE

Although getting chronologically older is inevitable, your body need not "age" as rapidly as is considered "normal." Most of the signs of aging—a sagging body being the most visible—are really the signs of an underused body. Hardening of arteries and lowering of lung capacity, for example, are likewise symptoms of an underused body. As years pile on, gravity does take its toll by compressing the spine and pulling muscles in a downward direction. That's why it's advisable for a sedentary man, whatever his birth date, to start working out. Through exercise, it's actually possible for a man to become biologically "younger" to the extent that he can improve his fitness and extend his longevity. In the process, he'll also *look* younger.

Of course, some fellows are going to have an easier time maintaining a youthful appearance than others. Weight is the biggest culprit. Even on otherwise slender individuals, fat has a way of depositing itself on the waist, hips, thighs, upper arms, and shoulder blades during middle age. Underworked muscles go slack all over. Consequently, anyone with a propensity to put on pounds easily—which particularly means anybody with an endomorphic frame, inclined toward burliness—must be especially diligent in working out. Yet fellows born with other body types aren't in for a free ride, since time's progress will progressively erode their inherent advantages.

The older one becomes, the wiser it is to concentrate on exercises to augment flexibility as a logical defense against the inclination of joints and muscles to stiffen. Exercising the heart and lungs likewise takes logical priority over building muscle mass. However, if one has worked oneself up to a good degree of fitness prior to middle age, there's no reason this healthy individual can't sustain a total system of exercise throughout his lifetime.

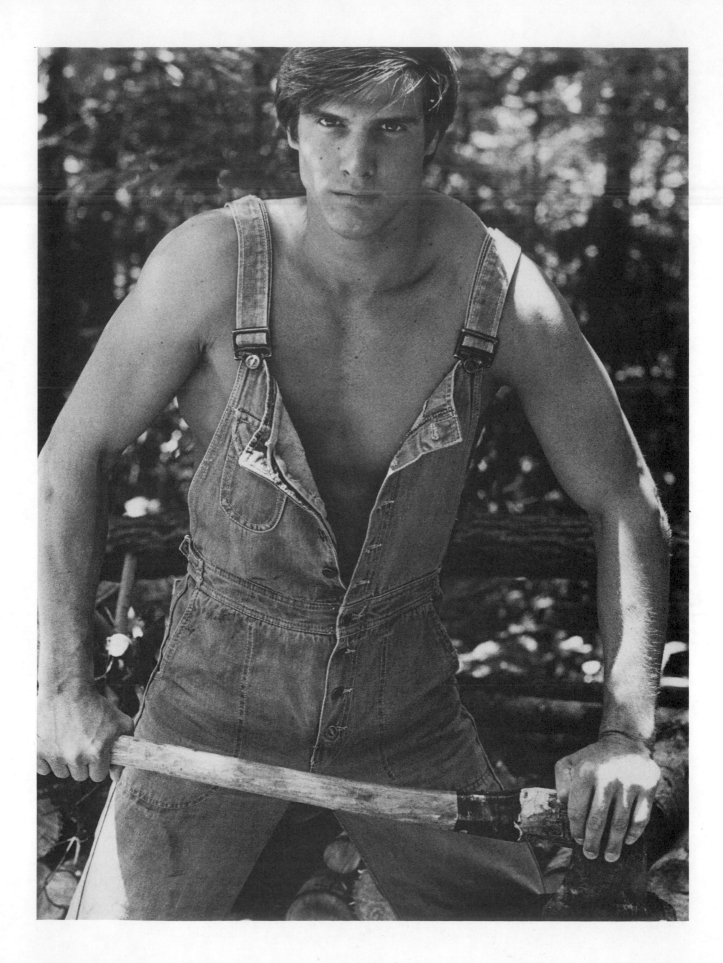

STRESS

Mental and emotional tension are not independent phenomena. When you're under stress, not only do you feel anxious; your body responds to your anxiety as well by tightening your muscles and accelerating your heartbeat. Both these responses can be alleviated by working out—although, of course, it's preferable to eliminate the source of anxiety. Easier said than done. But if you don't reduce stress when it comes your way, you're in deep trouble, potentially dangerous physical trouble.

Here's what your body does with anxiety. Muscular tension is only one barometer that life is getting to be too much for you to take calmly. When stress strikes, your brain (via the autonomic—a high-toned medical way of saying automatic—nervous system, over which you have no conscious control) tells your body that it's being threatened and to prepare for a siege. In self-defense, hormones are released that put the body on edge.

All this would be very helpful if events dictated that you actually had to physically defend yourself. But this mechanism isn't so hot if you don't dissipate your "flight-or-fight" instincts through action. When there is no actual confrontation to resolve the would-be peril and the feeling of stress continues, your body remains keyed up, adversely affecting the cardiovascular system . . . and your sense of well-being . . . and your muscle flexibility. Inflexible muscles are wasteful in two ways. First, energy is used to keep them constricted and that's energy that could be more properly channeled elsewhere. Second, tight muscles slow down the effective response of that whole area of the body, retarding efficiency. Also, tight muscles are more prone to injury.

Any type of exercise helps to dispel stress, but particularly helpful are types that incorporate repetitious, rhythmic movements. Meditation is also effective.

As the stress syndrome proves, physical fitness is highly influenced by emotional contentment. Seeking harmony of mind is as high-ranking as seeking harmony of body. Fortunately, in many ways the two pursuits can coincide.

WEIGHT

Transporting too many pounds on your frame is unhealthful because your heart is forced to work harder than if you weighed less just to keep you mobile. But poundage isn't the sole concern.

Picture two men—let's call them Howie and George—with the same build (they're both mesomorphs), height (5 feet 10, give or take a fraction), and weight (they both tip the scale at about 180). Howie looks sloppy with his paunch, while George looks dynamic with his expansive chest. The difference is in the amount of fat versus muscle each guy is carting. And that difference explains why Howie, whose extra weight is derived from fat, is far less fit than George, whose pronounced musculature contributes significantly to his well-being. Howie is overweight; George isn't.

Body fat represents about 18 percent of the "average" man's total weight. But an "average" marathon runner's body may contain only 10 percent body fat or less. How you work out affects these percentages. Lifting weights is far less effective in reducing body fat than is running or skipping rope, simply because the latter actions burn up more energy.

Body fat doesn't contribute to muscular strength. Food provides calories to fuel the body. But when calories consumed are insufficient to do the stoking, the body burns up some of its own fat, thereby decreasing its stored-up supply when requiring extra energy during a workout. So while exercising per se doesn't really cause you to lose weight (depending upon your diet, you can—and may want to—gain weight while exercising vigorously), whenever food intake is diminished and physical activity is heightened, you will reduce body fat while simultaneously building up your body.

Because of his genetic propensity toward stringiness, it's easiest for the ectomorph to lose weight while working out, even if it's poundage he wants to keep. Similarly, a sinewy mesomorph will drop weight more readily than an endomorph, who is naturally inclined toward weight gain and a burly appearance. As a result, an endomorph whose goal is weight control through exercise must partake heavily of activities that call for sustained effort. Running on a treadmill or riding a mechanical bicycle—or doing the real things—is especially helpful, as are sprinting, rowing, racquet sports, and swimming.

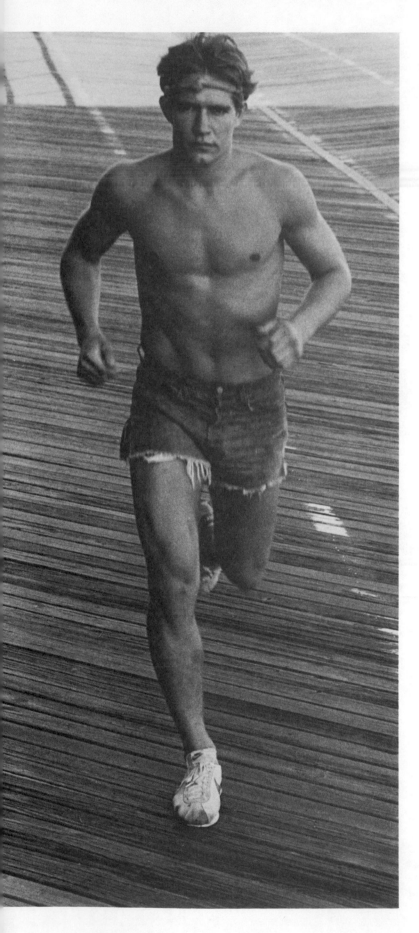

Test. You're asked to see how much distance you can cover in any combination you concoct of walking, running, and jogging (even crawling, if that's all you feel like doing at closing time) during twelve minutes. To earn an excellent rating, no matter how you accomplish it as long as you don't thumb a ride, you must traverse at least a mile and three-quarters. Less than a mile is deemed very poor, while anywhere between a mile and a quarter and a mile and a half is considered fair.

The drawback of this method is that it tests only aerobic fitness. Another shortcoming is that someone in really bad shape shouldn't even attempt to take the test.

That's the real hang-up in any self-proctored fitness analysis. If you're really healthy (if not necessarily wealthy and wise) and already blessed with a high degree of aerobic fitness, you won't come into harm's way during the testing rituals. But if you're not anywhere near a glorious or even an average condition, you could be asking for trouble while innocently trying to gauge your own fitness level.

AEROBIC FITNESS

Remembering these words of warning, if you want to administer your own test for aerobic fitness, see how long it takes you to trot-dash-walk-run-jog-skip-amble-sprint-or-otherwise-travel a mile and a half. Make sure the ground you'll cover is level.

Since your aim is to rate yourself, this isn't really a competition. The quest is for information, not praise. On the other hand, for the test to have any meaning you need to score your performance.

If you require fifteen minutes or more to cross the finish line, admit your display was poor.

If you can complete the course in about twelve or thirteen minutes (give or take a few seconds), call your exploit average—which is really pretty good, since not too many guys can match the score.

If you make it in eleven minutes or less, your tour-de-force feat is truly excellent.

But there's more to the test than the distance. With enough sheer determination and moxie, you might be able to cover the course in eleven minutes only to collapse in a heap. That is no sign of excellence.

Your heart's reaction during the deed is essential to the test finding. When you're through, if your pulse is dangerously near your maximum safe heartbeat, your aerobic fitness is definitely not excellent. On the other hand, if your heart is pumping at only 60 percent of maximum capacity, then you undoubtedly deserve an excellent grade.

No foolproof formula exists to correlate your time

for completing the track with your concluding pulse rate. Use your own common sense. Theoretically, if you take fifteen minutes to round out the territory, you get only a poor rating. But if your pulse is not much higher at the end than at the beginning, obviously you aren't giving the course a sincere try. Working a bit more strenuously, you could probably achieve an average score.

However, if your face is turning tomato red while you're undergoing this test and your chest is heaving like a bellows, for heaven's sake, stop. Face facts: Friend, you need more time before any contemplation of vigorous exercise. Build up your aerobic fitness first, slowly and comfortably to ensure long-lived results. (You'll be told how to do so safely in Chapter 8.)

And never forget while taking any fitness test that you should always stop at the earliest sign of ache or pain, especially in the chest: You're only trying to ascertain the shape you're in; trying to "prove yourself" by straining beyond your limit only proves you're foolhardy.

FLEXIBILITY FACTOR

Don't those two words sound good and look nice? It's too bad they don't have a very precise meaning.

If you can give contortionists a run for their money by tying yourself into a pretzel, you're flush with the flexibility factor. If you can't bend to tie your shoelaces, you're totally lacking in it.

How can you test your flexibility? By stretching all muscles to their absolute limit. That involves pain. Not the best solution.

So that you won't rue your ruthlessness tomorrow, take care with this test.

Seated on the floor, legs about a foot apart in front of you, extend your arms straight up over your head. Slowly stretch your hands toward your toes while bending forward from the waist.

If you can comfortably touch your fingertips to your toes, do so. If you can't, *don't*; just point your fingers toward those digits. Conversely, if you can easily touch your toes, can you clasp your feet with your hands and comfortably hold the position for fifteen seconds?

Now, even if your fingers won't extend to your toes, reach as close to them as you can and tuck your chin toward your chest. (If you *can* touch your toes or clasp your feet, that's what you should do before tucking your chin.) With an arch in your back, lower the top of your head toward your knees, but *don't strain yourself unduly*.

With minimum discomfort, can you lower your head to within twelve inches of your knees? Within six inches? Can you rest your head against your knees?

Obviously, the farther you can stretch and tuck, the higher is your flexibility factor. Also obviously,

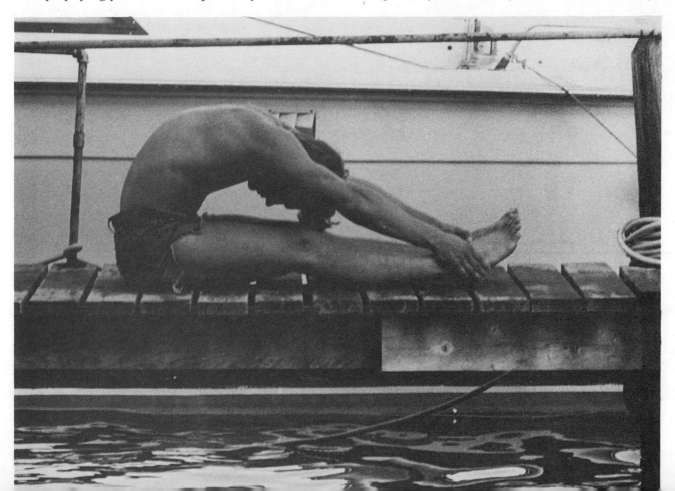

if you jam yourself into a position your muscles aren't prepared to assume, you're going to be sorely sorry.

If you can't complete the toe-touch and your head bobbles more than a foot from your knees when you tuck yourself forward, score the execution as poor.

If you're able to touch your toes but can't clasp your feet, and if your head will come about six inches or so from your knees but no closer, rate your performance as average—which is really damn good.

If you can clasp your feet and touch your head to your knees, why do you need this book? That's a first-rate, excellent job.

Appraise your pulse, of course.

Although this routine doesn't challenge the flexibility of all your muscles, it qualifies as an indicator for overall agility.

Odds are the farther you can stretch and tuck, the more gracefully you'll accomplish the feat, since coordination and flexibility usually intertwine. Practice affects coordination too. As you repeat body motions over and over again, your body "memorizes" the routine, performing it more easily and fluidly with time. Practice makes for perfected flexibility and coordination. Those two join forces for a state of grace.

STRENGTH SYNDROME

Another nice phrase, right? And also less than definitive.

Your strength is difficult to put a finger on because it also involves endurance.

In terms of measurable strength, the more pounds you can lift, the stronger you are. If your cardiovascular system is also strong, you gain in endurance.

To get a general gauge of your strength, see how many push-ups you can perform. It's not the most accurate test, since who's to say which will cause you to give up first, your muscles or your cardiovascular system? On the other hand, can you suggest a better way?

Once again, the reason for this test isn't to claim the title of push-up champ of all time. If you strain and struggle and subject yourself to inordinate stress, you'll be proclaiming that you're the chump of all time. Got it?

If you can't complete ten push-ups, judge your performance poor.

If you come out near twenty, call it an average effort, which is far from bad.

If you count off more than thirty push-ups, count your achievement excellent.

Don't forget to temper these ratings with a consideration of your heartbeat at the conclusion of the task.

There's one more problem with this test: It doesn't measure the strength of all your muscles. Well, no test is perfect. At least it roughly indicates your strength as a guideline for use later on.

Just for the fun of it, if you've got a chinning bar handy, you could take another strength test to see

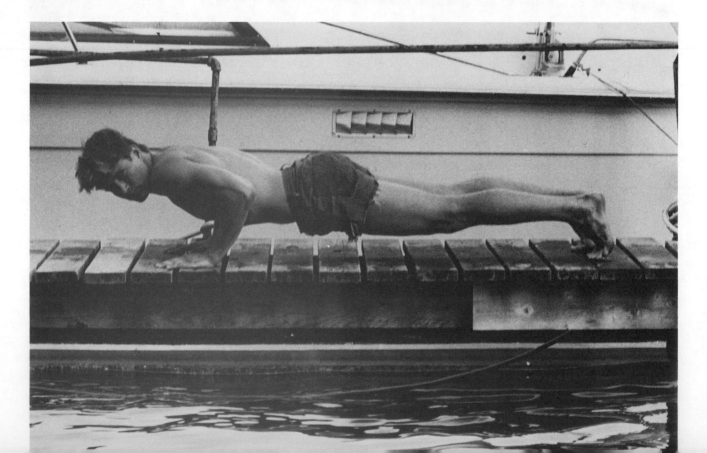

how the results stack up against the push-up rating. To make sure the results are worth comparing, don't take this one after completing your push-ups. Wait until you're well rested and your muscles have regrouped.

If you can't complete five chin-ups, sorry, that's poor.

If you can do eight or ten, good, that's a solidly average showing.

If you can do more than twelve, fine and dandy, that's excellent.

Need you be reminded to check your pulse when you're through to see what it's up to?

One more time: This entire series of tests to check out your present level of all-around fitness is designed only to do precisely that—to help you rate yourself right now. You can't pass or fail. All you can do is learn. However, if you soar through them with flying colors, you'll be able to jump right in at an intermediate, or even an advanced, level for your particular body type—*when* the time comes to start working out. Just as you had to have an overall fix on your performance level in *all* areas before taking the plunge, you still need to know a little more specific exercise data. So, onward.

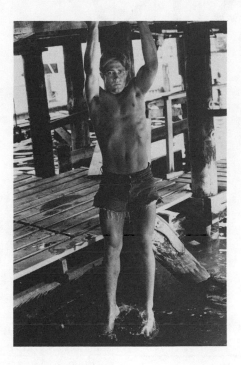

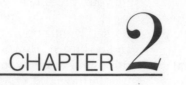

BASIC TRAINING

BUILDING BLOCKS

Did you know that some football coaches recommend ballet lessons to their backfield? Or that a long-distance runner may lift weights as an integral part of his training?

Do you know why?

If you read what was implicit between the lines in the previous chapter, you already have the answer. To spell it out more explicitly: No one sport or exercise ever works out the body to its fullest. To work yourself to your fittest—and most attractive—physical potential, you must participate in a variety of physical activities.

TUNING EXERCISE

These imperative movements are usually called *warm-ups.* They prepare the body for stepped-up exertion. Without them, you run the risk of injury as soon as you're under way.

Each and every time you exercise, no matter how conscientiously careful you try to be, some damage is done to muscle tissue. As your muscles heal themselves, they shorten . . . which reduces their flexibility and sets them up for another injury. However, as muscles become warmer, they also become more pliable. The best muscle warmer is your own circulation. And how do you increase this blood flow? By exercise. But since you can't jump right into heavy exercise without hurting your muscles, you must exercise *slowly* at first to bring blood *slowly* to the muscles. *Several minutes of tuning exercises are mandatory prior to every exercise session—*which means, since you'll be exercising daily, that you'll be tuning up daily. (These movements are illustrated in Chapter 4.)

In addition to tuning your body for working out, warming up also helps cut down on soreness when

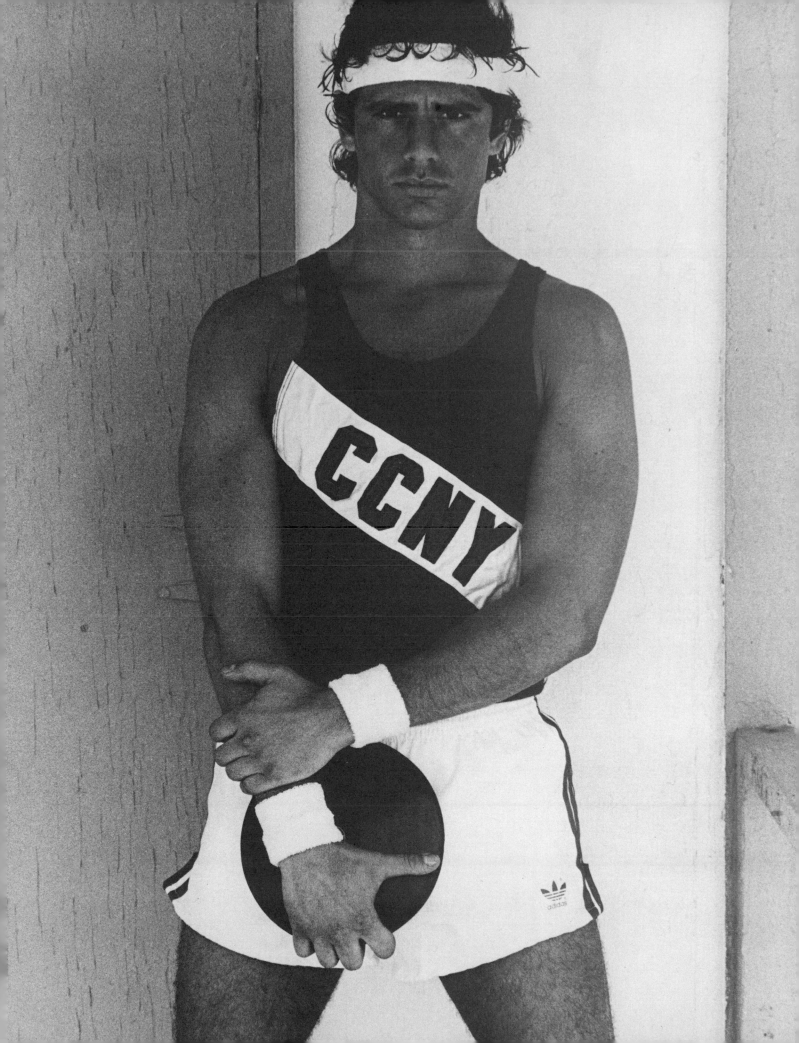

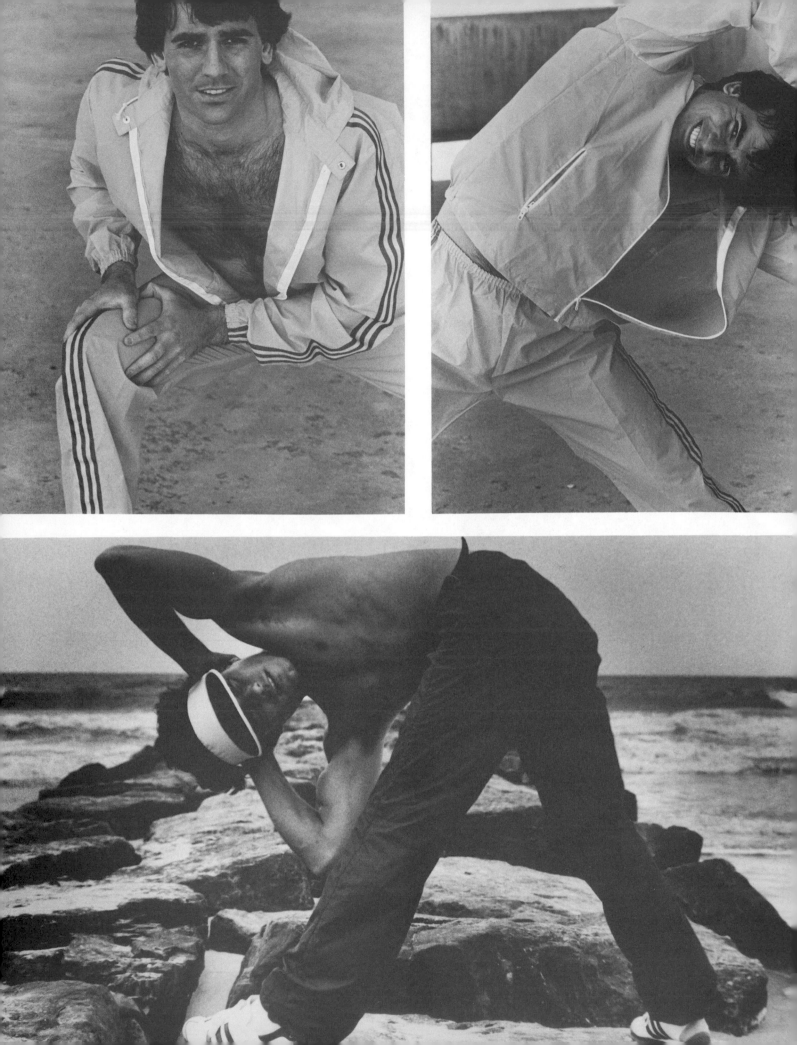

the session is completed. *All body types* require tuning exercises in equal amounts.

LIMBERING EXERCISE

This form of exercise is designed primarily to increase the mobility of the muscles, making them more flexible. Stretching is always involved, as in toe touching, for example.

Limbering exercises require precision, not speed, as good form is essential here. When properly executed, they help prevent injury to muscles and joints, and they are excellent for easing body tension.

Although limbering movements don't do much to improve the cardiovascular system or to increase muscle size, they are a requisite for strengthening muscles. This is why. A "muscle-bound" individual is someone who has concentrated on muscle mass and ignored stretching; as a consequence, his muscle/joint mobility has actually decreased, and so has his ability to use his pumped-up muscles for any practical purpose.

For best results, *limbering exercises should be performed daily.* (The movements are illustrated in Chapter 5.) Burly endomorphs will find that limbering exercises help build coordination, an attribute they often lack. Sinewy mesomorphs and stringy ectomorphs, already graced with higher levels of innate coordination, will improve their muscle mobility and heighten their overall physical performance.

The more limber your muscles are, the more they're primed to perform without strain. Cosmetically, limber muscles help a body appear graceful. In fact, a body can't be graceful if it isn't fluidly flexible.

MAINTENANCE EXERCISE

This type of exercise will maintain both your health and your endurance. You must prepare your body for maintenance exercise with tuning and limbering movements.

Depending upon your needs and your present physical shape, maintenance exercise incorporates several ways of working out.

Aerobic Exercise. The easiest way to comprehend the importance of aerobic activity is to compare it with its diametric opposite, *anaerobic* activity.

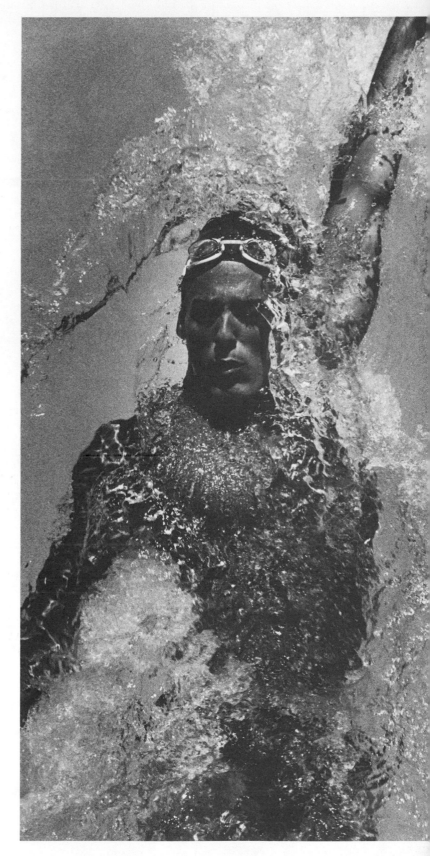

33

An anaerobic task is accomplished in a short burst of movement so rapid that the body is never called upon to seek additional oxygen to energize the deed, because your organism holds sufficient oxygen in reserve. A ten-second sprint is the epitome of anaerobic labor, since it can be executed without inhalation or exhalation. At the conclusion of the action, however, the body has an "oxygen debt"—which explains why sprinters gulp for air (oxygen) at sprint's end.

A fit body is up to the dramatic rigors of anaerobic labor; an unfit body isn't.

Enter aerobic exercise. Aerobic work is fueled by oxygen. But it does not create an "oxygen debt" because oxygen is replenished constantly during the labor itself via the act of breathing.

When the cardiovascular system is tip-top, the bloodstream supplies the body and muscles with sufficient oxygen and nutrients while spiriting away the waste—principally carbon dioxide, what's left of the air you breathe after it's metabolized—that's a by-product of exercise. Areas not engaged in the exercise lose some of their blood supply to the involved areas. The more efficient the cardiovascular system is, the longer this activity can go on without an undue rise in the heartbeat.

If you're near the top of your physical potential, not only do you have greater cardiovascular endurance, you can also safely handle sudden, strenuous activity of the anaerobic sort. Lacking in aerobic fitness, you shouldn't even try.

Aerobic exercise—any activity that uses large muscle groups (including the heart and lungs) rhythmically over a sustained period of time at a rate fairly much above your resting heartbeat but below your maximum safe heartbeat—is the surest way to maintain physical fitness . . . assuming you're already fit. If not, aerobic exercise (walking, running, rope skipping, cycling, and the like) is the surest way to become physically fit and then to maintain that fitness.

To keep its good benefits going, *aerobic exercise should be undertaken every* other *day for twenty to thirty minutes*.

Although some arguments can be made for daily aerobic exercise in special cases, this is just too much to ask of your body when other routines are added to work out the total organism—particularly if you lift weights. (*Aerobic and weight-lifting workouts should be done on an every-other-day basis, alternating aerobics one day with weight training on the next, then* *back to aerobics the next day, followed by weight training on the following day, and so on.*)

Although aerobic exercise can't be topped for contributions to cardiovascular fitness, generally it does little to alter the body aesthetically. In and of itself, it won't guarantee weight loss, nor will it build muscle. Even so, it is the framework on which any legitimate exercise regimen must be based. It sets the stage so the body can indulge in other types of activity that more effectively transform body dimensions.

All body types benefit from aerobic exercise, especially endomorphs that are inclined toward burliness. Their bodies often have a higher-than-average proportion of body fat, which strains their hearts. One salutary result of aerobic exercise is an increased number of capillaries in exercised muscles. This allows the body to use more oxygen and nutrients every minute. Similarly, blood flows more freely, tending to wash away fatty deposits. Red blood cells proliferate more readily, making the respiratory system more efficient. Some forms of high blood pressure are reduced.

Stringy-oriented ectomorphs naturally have more stamina, but an unexercised cardiovascular system won't keep regenerating itself. Thus, the need for aerobic exercise never diminishes. (Recommended aerobic exercises are found in Chapter 6.)

CALISTHENICS. Jumping jacks and sit-ups, examples of calisthenics you probably performed in adolescence, may or may not promote aerobic fitness. They don't if you dabble at them for a few minutes or so; they do if you keep going at them, nonstop, for half an hour. Although calisthenics can be directed toward aerobic purposes, they are usually employed to maintain muscular endurance and flexibility.

Depending upon how arduously you go into calisthenics, you get different results. That's because they're a form of what is called *isotonic* exercise. (Weight lifting is also an isotonic activity, but its goal is specifically to build new—not merely to maintain existing—muscle. More about that shortly.)

In general, isotonics have you put your muscles through a range of movements repetitiously. In calisthenics without equipment, external resistance is low—only the weight of your body. Therefore, when your muscles are in reasonable shape, although calisthenics affect strength, endurance, and coordination, they do a far better job at increasing

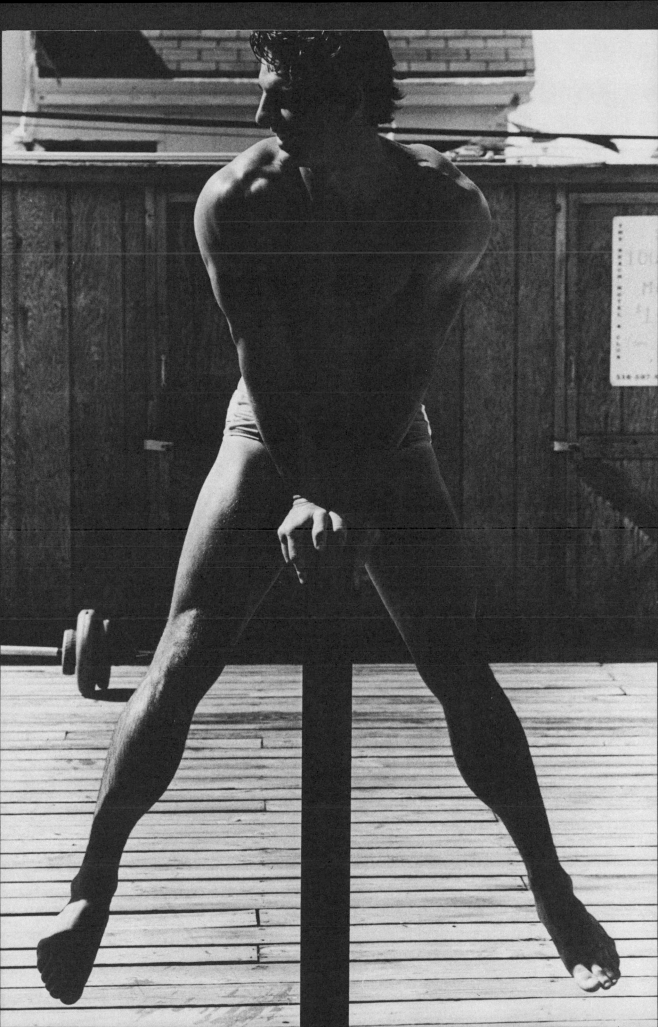

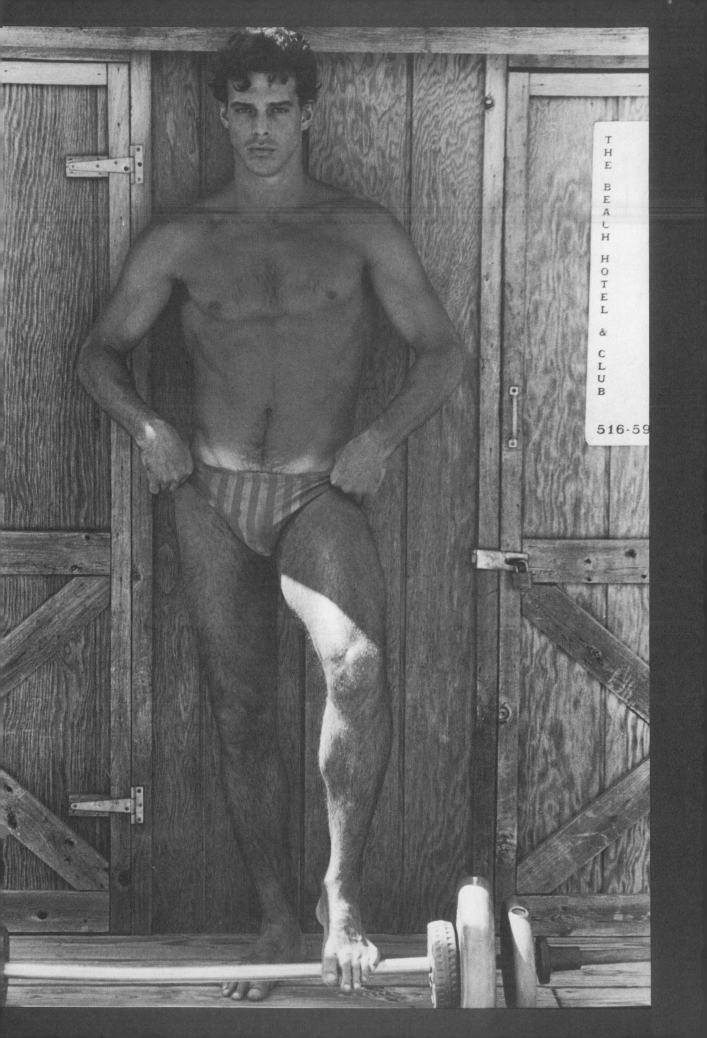

endurance and coordination than in raising your strength dramatically.

Meanwhile, building muscle endurance is not to be taken lightly. As you increase your muscular endurance, your muscles take oxygen from the blood more readily. When muscles tire less easily, they're more efficient in getting rid of waste. They don't feel as tired or sore after working out and heal more quickly. Conversely, fatigued muscles lose coordination and eventually stop performing altogether.

Per usual, burly guys have the most to gain from calisthenics.

BUILDING EXERCISE

This form of activity is aimed directly at your skeletal muscles, not your heart. It isn't really health-producing, only dimension-changing. But if the right preconditions are set, it is never unhealthful.

Technical jargon aside, muscles increase in size because they have been overworked. Your brain tells muscles to grow to handle a difficult job more easily the next time. The threadlike fibers within muscles thicken. The only way to make muscles grow is to exhaust them.

ISOMETRICS. These are static exercises. The idea is to tighten the muscles and to exert pressure against other fixed muscles or an immovable object. And that's it. The heart goes unexercised, but if aerobic exercise is performed in conjunction with isometrics, that's no problem.

But isometrics pose another problem. They don't pretend to be more than a shortcut method of building muscle mass. And they're difficult to monitor: You're supposed to resist harder and harder, but there's no real way to measure your effort as there is in weight training. Similarly, once muscles have been built, isometrics aren't very useful in creating still more muscle volume. They're best as therapy for people incapacitated by illness or injury for a lengthy period. Unless you're passionate about pushing against doorframes, you're better off ignoring isometrics entirely, heading straight into another type of building exercise, provided you have some degree of muscle strength to begin with. If you're a proverbial 90-pound weakling incapable of walking a block without palpitations, build cardiovascular endurance first.

RESISTANCE EXERCISES. Unlike isometrics, resistance exercises involve movement, though not oodles of it. When you lift a weight, your muscles

VISUALIZATION

Your imagination can help you shape up.

Think about your physical potential. In fact, do more than think about it: *Picture* it. Conjure up a mental image of how you will look when you've successfully worked out. Commit it deeply to memory.

You're indulging in the act of visualization. It's as if your imagination is affixing that picture of yourself within easy reach for reference and reassurance.

The more concretely you visualize how you will look, the more convinced you become about your ultimate achievements. A firm notion of where you're heading spurs you on. If this sounds a bit like self-hypnosis, that's because it is—believing is a requisite to achieving.

You should call to mind that picture of your eventual self periodically as you work out. With time's passage, notice how much more closely you are approximating that mental picture.

Only your imagination can photograph your potential physique, but to chart your progress, you can have a friend shoot you in your present shape. It should be a full-length photo, front view, with you in the briefest of brief attire to record as much of you as modesty allows. In fact, have rear and side views taken as well.

Once those photographs are developed, do some more visualizing. Superimpose your mental image of the you you'll become over the prints. Note what areas of your body require the most work. Visualize the precise changes in proportions that will take place.

While you're visualizing your attainments, don't become so immersed in fancy that you believe you've already reached the desired configuration. To give yourself an objective checkpoint, get a small notebook and record all your body measurements, from the size of your neck to the circumference of both calves. (It's easier if you have someone else wield the tape measure unless you're a contortionist.) Every three or four weeks, jot down your new body dimensions and go through another photo session to document your progress.

Before every exercise session, reinforce yourself by calling up that vision of the body you're creating. Don't dwell on negatives. Always think to the future, confident that it's only a matter of time before the you in the mirror looks exactly like the you inside your head.

Visualization really does help. Be a believer.

go through a series of movements, moving against the resistance of the weight.

A feather offers little resistance, so lifting a feather a thousand times won't increase muscle mass. Doing the same with a cement block is much harder. Lifting one a thousand times will definitely develop the arm muscles of someone who doesn't deal with cement blocks daily. It won't affect the musculature of a person who's been lifting two cement blocks regularly for a month or more.

Any type of body responds to resistance exercises, although sinewy mesomorphs adapt the quickest, stringy ectomorphs the slowest.

PROGRESSIVE-RESISTANCE EXERCISES. Once your muscles have become accustomed to specific resistance, unless you force them to work continuously without any rest so that the muscles are exhausted by the sheer amount of intensively extended labor, they won't increase in size until the resistance becomes greater. When it does, the muscles must once again work harder. The brain tells them to enlarge, and they do. Until they're so adept at handling that resistance that the resistance must again be increased.

Progressive-resistance exercises are an orderly progression of tasks to build muscle mass without harming yourself. (Suggested building exercises are illustrated in Chapter 7.) However, some "harm" is inevitable and even desirable, for without it, muscles will never enlarge. But too much of a harmfully "good" thing can be too much.

In a total exercise program, when your muscles are being challenged in several ways, progressive-resistance exercises should not be followed daily. A day of rest from this type of activity is called for if you're going to be up to the rigors of other routines—especially the physical demands of aerobics, performed on those days you are not involved in weight training.

Naturally, there are limits to the weight you can lift, so dimensional physical changes are also finite. However, odds are you are not seeking extravagant additions to your musculature. (If you are, you should be devoting yourself almost exclusively to weight training.) Once you have reached a desired body configuration, you would revert from progressive-resistance to fixed-resistance exercise to keep those contours.

COOLING EXERCISE

Soreness or stiffness following a workout happens because carbon dioxide and toxins released during exercise haven't worked their way out of the muscles yet. This can occur when you push your muscles farther than they're ready to be pushed, or when your cardiovascular system isn't working as well as it should. It can also occur when you stop a workout session earlier than you should: Just as you must warm up before starting to exercise, *you should always cool down before you're really and safely finished.* (Since you'll be working out daily, your every-day workout will incorporate tuning up, limbering, and *either* maintenance *or* building exercises on an every-other-day alternating basis, concluding with cooling exercises.)

Your heart busily pumps more blood to the muscles during a workout just like a loyal repeating machine, but it can't slow down as quickly as you can stop exercising. It will just go on working at its higher level for some time—and at some risk to you.

After fueling the muscles during exercise, blood must be refreshed in the heart and lungs on a return trip via the veins. The contracted muscles press the veins, aiding the blood's speedy return to the heart and lungs. Fine. But when the cessation of exercise is abrupt, muscles stop contracting. Not so fine. Blood is still being pumped to the muscle area, but it isn't being moved out at such a clip. Blood may "pool." Too much of it remains in one part of the body (especially the legs), causing a temporary shortage somewhere else (particularly in the brain). A feeling of faintness—or an out-and-out faint—may follow.

A slow reduction of exercise helps establish a more normal blood flow while simultaneously flushing out waste from the exercised muscles.

Since muscles tend to shorten during maintenance and building exercise, cooling exercise should incorporate limbering movements. (Cooling exercises are illustrated in the second half of Chapter 4.)

Every individual should conclude a workout with cooling exercises, regardless of body type or the type of activity.

SUMMARY

For optimal benefit, working out must be seen as a series of steps, each one setting the groundwork for the next.

To tune the body for the workout, warm-ups are a must.

After the body has started its tuning, limbering exercise should always follow. Stretched muscles

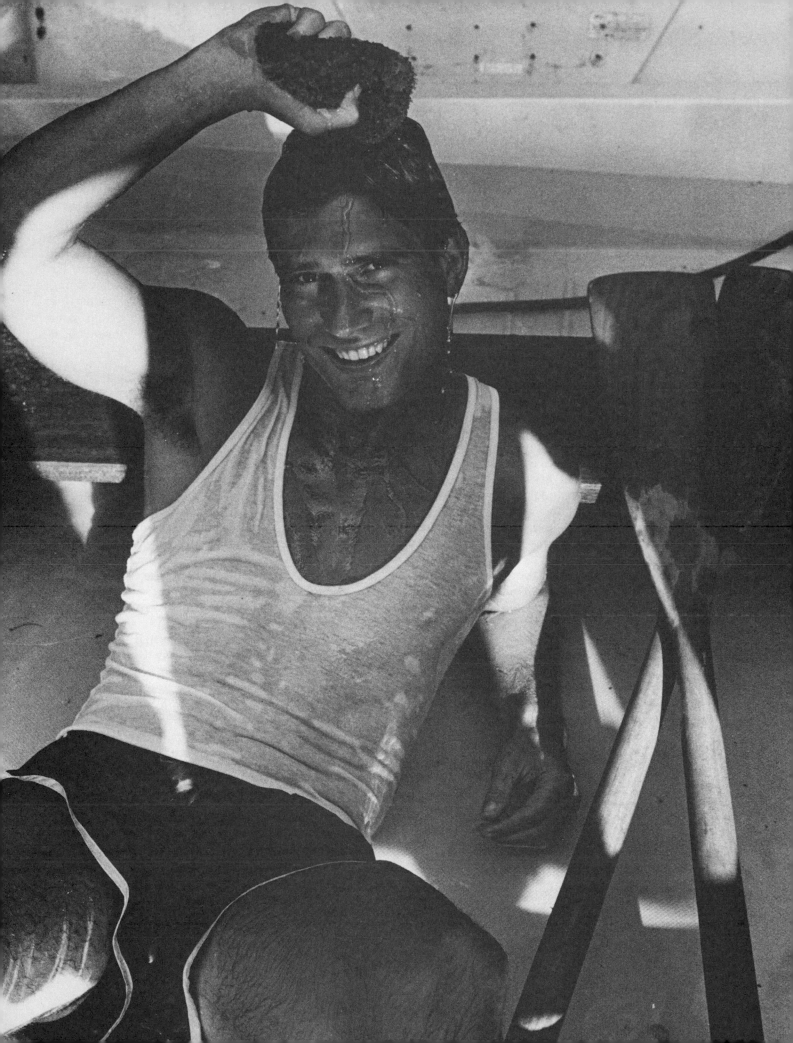

are more mobile. This increased flexibility makes the entire workout less hard on the body while promoting greater efficiency during the routines that follow.

Because aerobic fitness is the framework on which working out is built, maintaining cardiovascular endurance always has top priority. Once a program is progressing full-steam, however, it's physically more economical to stick to an every-other-day schedule of concentrated aerobic exercise.

Maintaining the organism also involves sustained muscular endurance. If you are interested only in retaining an already-achieved musculature, this too can be realized on an every-other-day schedule of fixed-resistance exercise, performed on those days you are *not* doing aerobics. (Calisthenics also do the trick.)

If you want to increase body dimensions and enlarge existing muscles, building exercises must be added to the regimen. These are among the most strenuous activities, since muscles must first be exhausted by overwork before they'll thicken. These exercises should not be performed daily, because the muscles will never have the opportunity to heal.

Whether a workout has been light or heavy, it must always be concluded with movements that cool down the body and reinstate a normal blood flow. The cool-down should include stretching exercises to reduce soreness and encourage muscle fluidity.

And since any form of exercise always subjects the body to a degree of wear-and-tear, your body must be primed again before undertaking another bout of working out.

And so the cycle revolves.

(Have the repetitions made it clear? In case they haven't, here's yet another reiteration: In a system of *total* exercise, you warm up and stretch daily; after limbering, you will proceed to either aerobic or resistance exercise, but not both on the same day; and you will end *every* daily workout with cooldowns.)

FUELING UP

It's hard to believe, but many people don't know how to breathe. Oh, they get air, or they wouldn't be walking about, but often they breathe so shallowly that they're rationing oxygen unnecessarily. The entire body requires oxygen, and any shortage affects the whole organism as well as one's emotional outlook.

While oxygen is always vital, during exercise it's even more critical. To get an adequate oxygen supply, you should breathe *deeply*, not from the chest, but from the diaphragm—*under* the chest, so that the diaphragm muscle lifts the rib cage when you inhale.

In practical terms, this means that during any form of exertion you should do what many people don't. Generally, you should inhale before initiating any physical activity, then exhale while performing the activity; you should *not* hold your breath, for that cuts off oxygen supply. Instead of breathing jerkily, you should breathe rhythmically. Imagine that you're pulling oxygen down through your lungs into your abdomen before slowly sending it back upward and out your nose.

Deep breathing not only supplies the body with a more ample oxygen supply. It also helps in the elimination of waste carbon dioxide which should not be left languishing in the lung recesses.

You can breathe deeply anytime, so when you exercise is less important than doing it right by following a regular schedule. Morning? Afternoon? Evening? It doesn't matter, provided you're reasonably rested and nourished to fuel your workout.

In theory, you *could* shuffle workout periods into open slots within each day's calendar. In practice, floating exercise timetables never pan out. An excuse invariably offers itself to postpone the workout for an hour or two; then, flash! the day is through and you're unexercised.

Working out requires commitment and concentration. Halfhearted efforts usually yield zero results. You should set aside from half to a full hour at the same time each day to devote totally and exclusively to exercise. You must free your mind as well as your appointment book: When you're preoccupied with matters other than keeping track of how your body responds during physical activity, you're not giving your all . . . and you're not getting your all out of the workout.

If your job is physically exhausting, obviously you shouldn't exercise at work's end. Your body won't be up to it. It's smarter to finish the job, refresh yourself with a nap, then work out. With a physically demanding occupation, take your labor-connected rigors into account when devising your workout strategies.

Don't forget that once the workout is over, you'll need extra time to make yourself presentable. If you plan a morning workout before heading for the job, for example, most likely you'll shower and shave after exercising. Plan accordingly. (For more about exercising/grooming considerations, see Part III, PRIDE & GROOM.)

When settling upon what span to set aside for exercise, choose a time you'll realistically stick to. If you hate rolling out of bed, don't opt for working out first thing in the morning. You'll hate the clock-radio and hate the workout experience.

Initially, a half-hour daily will definitely suffice. As you progress, however, you will want to invest more time. Only in rare or quite advanced instances will you ever consider giving more than one hour to an hour and a half a day to working out.

EXERCISE MYTHS

If it doesn't hurt, it doesn't help.

This is blatantly false. Although minimal soreness is inevitable, it should be only that—minimal. Exercise is not torture. Too much pain indicates improper execution.

Strenuous exercise isn't good for you; it enlarges the heart and can cause heart attacks.

An oversized heart can be dangerous at birth, but increasing the heart's musculature through exercise is healthfully beneficial, since doing so increases its efficiency. Exercising beyond your capability can be hazardous, but as you increase your capacity for exercise, you simultaneously increase your physical fitness. It's less dangerous to work out at the proper pace than *not* to exercise.

When you stop exercising, muscle turns to fat.

No! Muscle is muscle, fat is fat, and that's that. It is true, however, that if you quit working out after shaping up, your muscles can lose their tone and power quite quickly. Putting on pounds is not automatic if you watch caloric intake. If a former exerciser doesn't adjust his eating habits and subsequently gains weight, he faces a quandary. He shouldn't diet without starting to exercise again. Dieting without exercising, he'll lose muscle as well as weight. Why? Because muscle isn't weightless, just fatless. Although fat is the *first* weight to go, on a crash diet with no exercise, weight is soon dropped from muscle too. Muscle demands activity to keep generating itself. When muscles get smaller, they weigh less.

More positively, degenerating worked-out muscles can do a fast about-face: By renewing his workouts, a former exerciser can shape up again in a shorter time than it takes someone who has never exercised to get into comparable shape.

Exercising makes you eat more, so you become fatter.

Actually, the reverse is often true. A good workout tends to curb the appetite. Certain individuals, however, do eat more—and should. Increased activity can trigger a need for increased food consumption to fuel the exercise. When a person works out correctly, the calories are burned off and don't add fat. It is possible to gain weight in muscle, the end result being that someone will look trimmer even if he weighs more.

Never drink water after exercising.

Wrong. So much water is expended during an arduous workout that your body craves fluids. Gulping down huge quantities of water could make you feel nauseated, but sipping a small amount is recommended. After half an hour or so, drink a couple of tall glasses of fluid.

Always take salt tablets when exercising in hot weather.

Terrible advice. During any steady workout, even in cool temperatures, you do sweat a lot, but losing salt is less serious than popping salt tablets indiscriminately into your system. A misdirected person who overuses them may cause his blood pressure to rise temporarily. With prolonged overuse, the blood pressure will stay artificially elevated for a prolonged time, courting heart attack. Salt tablets are counterproductive during exercise because they pull water normally located in the muscle tissue into the stomach to cut down the resulting salinity. This increases the possibility of dehydration. Salt lost through exercise is easily replaced at the next meal. But it's more pressing to replace water: Perspiration is composed of much more water than salt, so trying to retain salt at the expense of dehydration is nonsensical.

In only a few minutes a day, you can be physically fit.

Hogwash. No instant panaceas exist for physical fitness. Only an ongoing regimen combining limbering, maintenance, and building exercise will help you realize your physical potential. If you schedule only a couple of minutes of exercise a day, you're wasting your time.

Sex and exercise don't mix.

Whoever is responsible for spreading this pernicious rumor should be horsewhipped. Think about it. What's more breathtaking than good sex? And what's a more enjoyable way of building physical endurance? Sex and exercise are more than compatible; sex is the perfect adjunct to exercise because each one improves the other.

SLEEP

The healthful benefits of working out can be undone by lack of sleep. Sleep releases stress and relaxes muscles, revitalizing them so they can face the rigors of a new day. Naturally, the better condition muscles are in before sleep, the greater will be sleep's rejuvenating power. On the other hand, lack of proper sleep means the muscles aren't restored. In fact, muscles become more, not less, tense without satisfying sleep. At first muscular coordination is only slightly lessened, but long bouts with sleeplessness will seriously hamper coordination.

On the positive side, exercise generally makes deep sleep easier to come by. And the positive effects of deep sleep are many. Although the body is relaxed, it is also working to restore and replace any damaged tissue.

No set formula exists for the amount of sleep an adult male requires, but seven and a half hours is usually adequate. Sleep induced by sleeping pills, however, tends not to be especially restful. Paradoxically, this is because drug-induced sleep is so deep that it suppresses the dreaming stage, and denied this kind of sleep for too long, someone can become an emotional wreck. So resorting to sleeping pills often leaves one feeling wrung out, not refreshed, the morning after.

You need nourishment to exercise, but not a stomach filled with food. Generally, it's best not to have eaten for about two hours before working out. (During heavy exercise, when large muscle groups are exerted, blood must be diverted from the stomach and intestinal tract to these areas. If too much undigested food is in the stomach, nausea or vomiting is likely.) Since thorough digestion takes a great deal longer than an hour or two, even when you do chow down a couple of hours prior to exercise, the nutrients you'll mostly be utilizing during the workout are derived from what you've eaten ten to twelve hours before the actual exertion. *That* food intake, then, is what fuels your workout, not what you've nibbled most recently.

Your body isn't very choosy about the type of food it uses to energize a workout; it calls upon whatever fuel is available. However, some foods are more quickly and easily utilized by your body while working out.

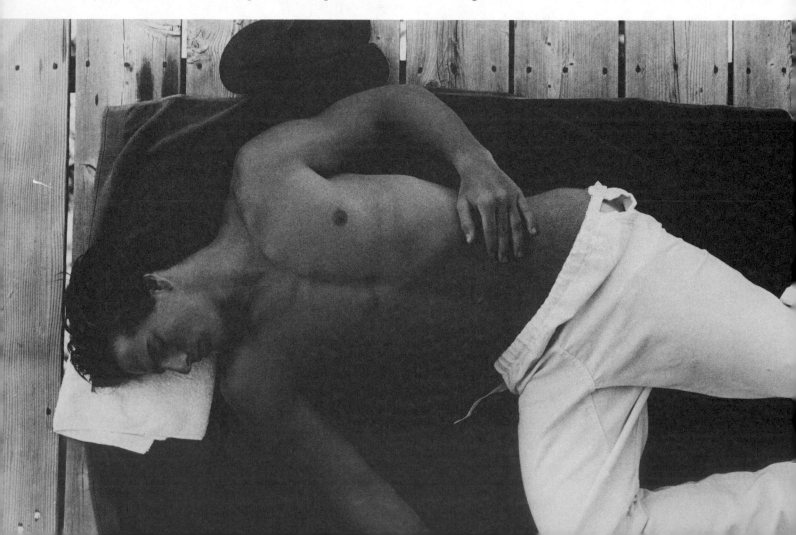

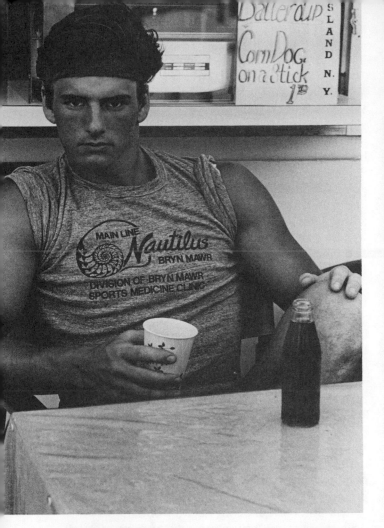
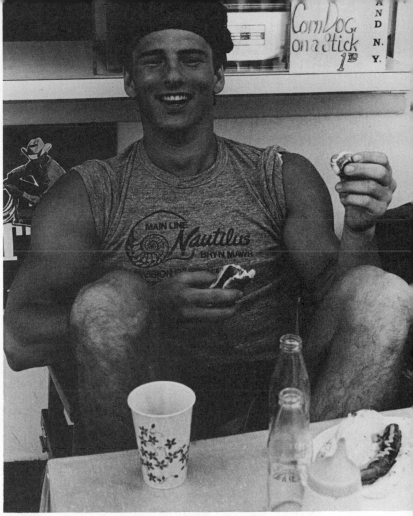

VITAMINS

Vitamins help the body utilize food. In a strict sense, they don't provide energy or build the body up. They only set the stage for good body performance when they're released during food digestion, at which time they're absorbed into the bloodstream.

Once vitamins (which never exist freely in the body anyway) get into the blood, they work to convert protein, carbohydrates, and fats into new tissue and new energy.

What this all means is that without food intake, vitamins are essentially useless: A diet consisting solely of vitamins or vitamin supplements is a sure route to starvation. They're only catalysts to keep food nutrients going, speeding up the chemical reactions in the organism.

Since the body cannot manufacture most vitamins, they must come from an outside source. Food is the best source. A well-balanced diet should provide all vitamins necessary.

If you follow the Food and Drug Administration's guidelines for recommended daily allowance (U.S. RDA) of the twelve classified vitamins, you can't go far wrong, provided you get 100 percent of the recommended nutrition.

Smoking greatly reduces vitamin C levels, so smokers should take this into account. A large intake of C supplements isn't hazardous, although kicking the habit is smarter. But ingesting large doses of C won't correct any damage through smoking to the cardiovascular system. Alcohol steals B vitamins, so drinkers should stock their bodies with B-complex supplements. But that won't prevent the development of liver damage. And a damaged liver interferes with vitamin absorption from even healthful foodstuffs.

Indiscriminate popping of fad vitamin pills can be detrimental rather than beneficial. Don't forget, vitamins do *not* make for stronger or more durable muscles, nor do they in and of themselves provide energy or build muscles. Wholesome food is a far better bargain than a bottle of vitamin capsules.

Contrary to a popular misconception, eating a candy bar a half-hour or so before exercising doesn't give you a rush of useful energy. Ingested sugar enters the bloodstream quickly. When you wolf down a gooey goody, the rapid sugar entry stimulates insulin to clear the new sugar out of the blood as fast as possible. When you're fairly sedentary, you experience a sort of energy "high" from the candy. But exercise automatically decreases the sugar level in the blood. When insulin, in conjunction with exercise, eliminates even more sugar, the blood-sugar level can drop too low, causing dizziness, poor coordination, and bad performance.

If you eat a candy bar during exercise, the results aren't much better. For one thing, it adds a lump in the gut. For another, to dilute the concentrated sugar, your body sends fluids to the stomach, drawing them from other body areas (where the fluids would be more useful) and making the stomach bloat, causing discomfort. The sugar from the candy bar does eventually get absorbed, but not soon enough to really help during the workout.

Another misconception is that a good steak a few hours prior to a workout is a good source of quick energy. Although protein is invaluable in building tissue, it isn't swell preceding exercise. Protein (especially meat protein) isn't easily digestible. Similarly, the fat in meat is slow to be digested. The longer it takes for food to be digested, the less efficient it is as fuel. Another drawback of protein as an energy source is that the body doesn't store it. When sated with protein, the body merely eliminates any extra.

Carbohydrates—both sugar and starch—are the best sources of energy when eaten at the right time. Sugars are absorbed easily and directly into the organism, but starches must first be digested. (Fruits and fruit juices are sugar-rich carbohydrates; pasta and potatoes are starch-rich carbohydrates.) Carbohydrates are stored in the muscles (as muscle sugar) and blood (as blood sugar), so energy is always immediately available. For this reason, carbohydrates are the preferred exercise food, although a well-rounded diet is always recommended.

The food you eat affects how ably you work out, but no foodstuffs turn into muscle more readily than any others. How conscientiously you work out is the ultimate factor in shaping up.

From the standpoint of energy efficiency, optimally your body should always be digesting food. To accomplish this, several small meals a day are preferable to two or three larger ones. From the standpoint of weight control, however, it doesn't matter when or how often you eat; the day's tally of total calories determines whether you lose or gain pounds.

And don't forget about good ol' water.

Even when not exercising, you require an intake of at least a quart and a half of fluids daily, since water is the body's largest single component and constantly needs replenishing. During exercise, an additional supply of water is called for to control your temperature and to keep your blood flowing at a good pace.

Thirst is usually not a reliable indication of the need for fluids, because once you've reached the point of being thirsty, your fluid level is already lower than desirable. Since a great deal of water is expended during a vigorous workout, you should drink two or three glasses of fluid an hour or two before beginning.

Failure to drink sufficient water (or juice) *before* exercising is doubly risky, because once you've begun working out your body absorbs fluids less easily than when you're mainly inactive. While it's not detrimental to drink during exercise—in fact, if your workout is longer than twenty minutes, you should—swallowing too much liquid at one time that isn't readily absorbed leaves you with a sloshy feeling.

If your kidneys are functioning properly—and if you have easy access to a urinal—there's no way

REVERSIBILITY

Fitness is an ongoing process. The cold truth is that even the most splendid physical specimen is less splendid if he stops working out for only a few weeks. This forlorn phenomenon is called *reversibility*. It first affects the cardiovascular system, which is why aerobic exercise is a lifelong commitment.

Eventually, when you don't work out as you should, you're not as successful with anaerobic efforts either. Initially, you'll be as strong as ever, but if you drop off muscle-building tasks even slightly, strength will diminish too. And your muscles will tell you so: For no apparent reason, they'll feel sore. But eventually the reason will be apparent: Your muscles will be shrinking, and the compression causes the pain.

The cruel lesson is that it takes a lot less time to get out of shape then to work up your fitness.

you can drink too much water. What your body doesn't use it just flushes out. On the other hand, drinking too little liquid can be downright harmful.

Dehydration causes several unpleasantries. All bodily reactions are slowed down, meaning new tissue isn't produced and energy isn't properly channeled. Without water to cool the body via perspiration, the internal temperature rises too high. Wastes aren't washed out of the bloodstream. Blood volume is actually decreased, so less oxygen and nutrients are available. Muscles weaken and you feel pooped.

To repeat: If you don't belly up to the water fountain before working out, you're asking for trouble.

The longer and more arduously you exercise, the more water you must consume during the workout itself. You'll probably end up with a fluid debit when you're finished anyway.

Ice water is *not* bad for you during exercise. In fact, cold fluids are better than warm ones. Ice water (or an iced drink) is absorbed faster, so it cools you faster too.

Cramps result from gulping too much water of any temperature, so it's wiser to take several small sips instead of one big belt.

If you don't need to relieve your bladder shortly after completing a workout, you haven't drunk enough fluids before or during the session.

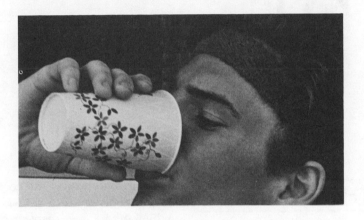

CHAPTER 3

LOCKER BOOM

ALONE/TOGETHER

The conundrum that puzzles every guy intent upon working himself into better shape is: To gym or not to gym?

If you're going to spend hard-to-come-by bucks on a gym (or health-club) membership, how can you be certain you'll get your money's worth? Usually you can't.

Does this mean you should simply choose a gym (or club) at random and hope for the best? Not at all. But you must be very thoughtful before joining any establishment. Remember, that paper you affix your signature to is a binding legal contract. Maybe you don't really want to be bound.

Surprisingly, your desired body configuration is of little concern when you're weighing the gym or at-home option. After all, your muscles aren't awfully discriminating. Your biceps won't notice whether you work out with barbells (in or out of a gym), at a real or mechanical rowboat, or at a gleaming (or rusty) machine within a swank (or seedy) spa. If you do it right, you'll end up with bigger biceps however you exercise.

Base your join-or-not decision on your personality makeup, not on your physical aspirations. Here are a few points to ponder.

Some fellows find the communal aspect of working out in a gym a boost to their concentration, while others are distracted. How are you more likely to respond?

Certain guys freeze up when they think others are watching, whereas less inhibited sorts are oblivious. What about you?

A man reluctant to ask for help or counsel will never receive equal attention from an instructor if a more aggressive type is on the premises. Will you make certain you receive the individual guidance your membership dues supposedly guarantee?

Try to imagine yourself in the gym milieu. If you're an independent loner or tend to be insecure, joining up may not be for you. Conversely, if you enjoy group interaction, signing on the dotted line could be a good move.

Even if your personality is suited for gym membership, look to your current physical condition. If you're in really poor shape, consider postponing gym activity until you can participate more confidently. When your abilities are far below the level of other members, it's easy to become discouraged and quit.

Look to your finances, too. If you join a gym, you're spared the expense of purchasing your own exercise equipment. A definite saving, right? Not so. Gym memberships must be renewed. Equip-

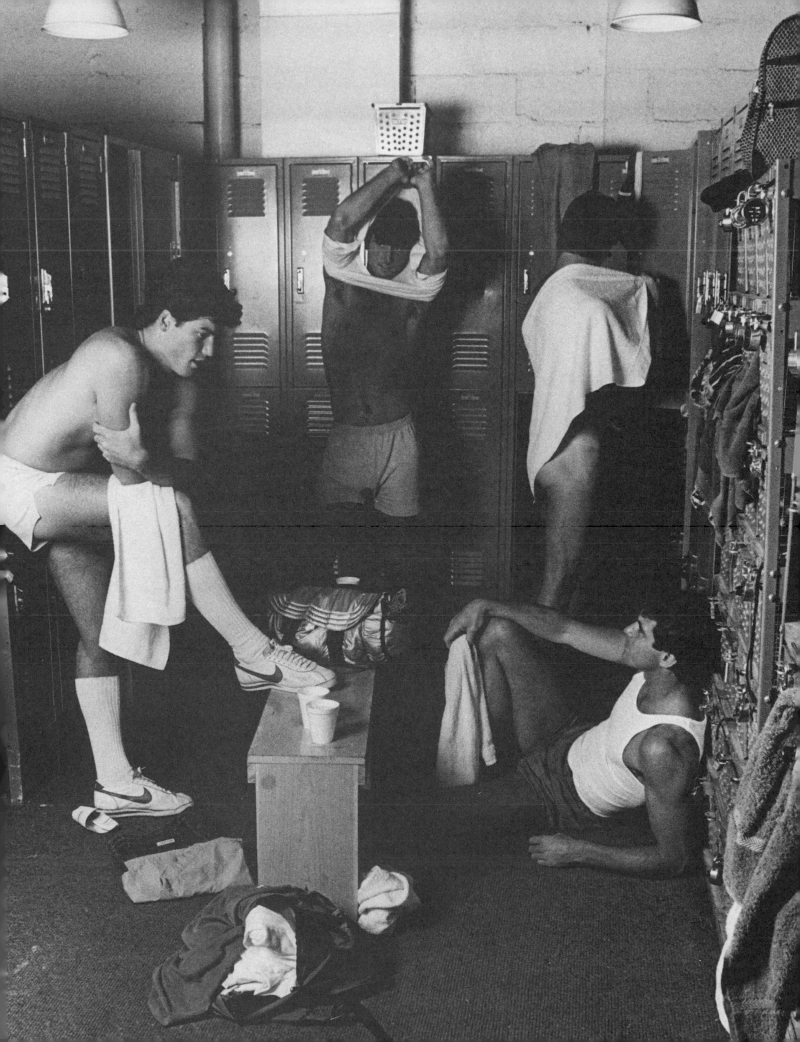

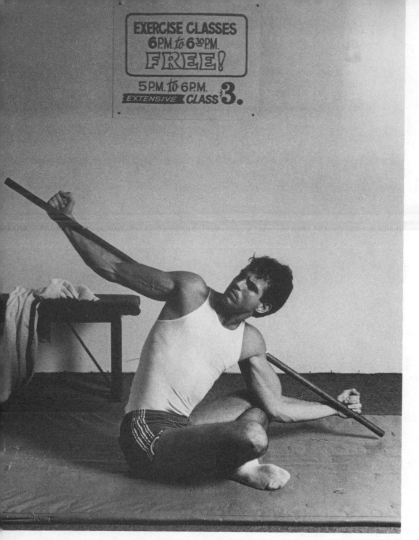

If you decide to forgo gym membership in favor of at-home workouts, a gym still has something invaluable to offer. Although most gyms and clubs will attempt to sell you annual memberships, sometimes you can maneuver a daily or weekly rate. If not, monthly rates are almost always available. Although these rates are proportionately higher than a year's membership, it's not a bad idea to secure a limited membership so you can learn the ropes of weight training before heading off on your own. If you try this ploy, be Machiavellian and play the innocent. Tell the manager you want to make certain you're up to lifting weights before committing to a full membership. You won't be given proper attention if he suspects you'll bolt the minute you've gotten your basic training.

Gyms are terrific for some types of fellows, terrific losses for others. Make sure you know which type you are.

ON THE TOWN

Say a gym is for you. What type of gym? Are you interested in an "old-fashioned" one with an odd lot of equipment to experiment with? Do you want

ment you purchase is yours for life without any strings attached (unless you buy it on credit). In the long run, buying the basic tools for working out at home can be cheaper than gym membership. *If you don't insist upon astronomically expensive paraphernalia.* Of course, you must have space in your abode to work out and to store the equipment.

One last thought. Consider what a gym does and doesn't offer. The main emphasis in most gyms (as opposed to exercise classes and centers that involve no use of equipment whatsoever) is on building muscle mass through progressive-resistance exercise. The gym helps you by providing equipment (which can be of various sorts) and, hopefully, by supplying an instructor to teach you perfect execution.

But there's more to working out than building muscle dimensions. For example, tuning, limbering, and maintenance exercises don't require specialized equipment, so there's no reason they must be done in a gym. Floor space is so limited at many gyms, in fact, that performing those activities may be frowned upon.

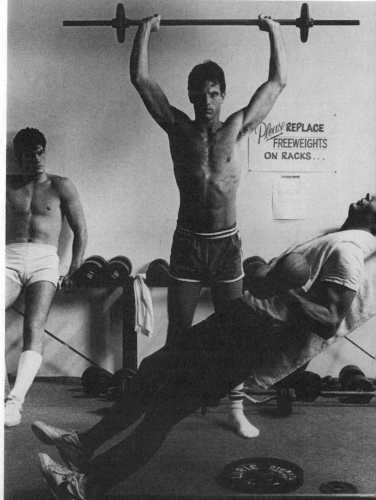

a facility specializing principally in weight training? Or are you inclined toward putting yourself in the mechanical hands of a Nautilus or Universal machine?

"Old-fashioned" gyms are numerically on the decline, being replaced by more streamlined establishments. Still, they have much to offer for first-time exercisers who want to try alternative methods of working out. Of course, as with all other gyms and clubs, the quality of individual enterprises varies greatly.

Gyms specializing in weight training come in good and poor varieties too, but more and more of them are opening, so it's fairly easy to find one to your liking. Since weight training is founded on the tenets of progressive-resistance exercise, you'll get this significant instruction if you gravitate to an establishment where the personnel themselves are well trained.

The Nautilus and Universal centers also focus on building muscle mass. Although their originators would ardently disagree, the visual differences attainable are negligible one from the other. Both systems of exercise rely on machines to put muscles through their paces. They are specifically designed for people who have an aversion to lifting weights

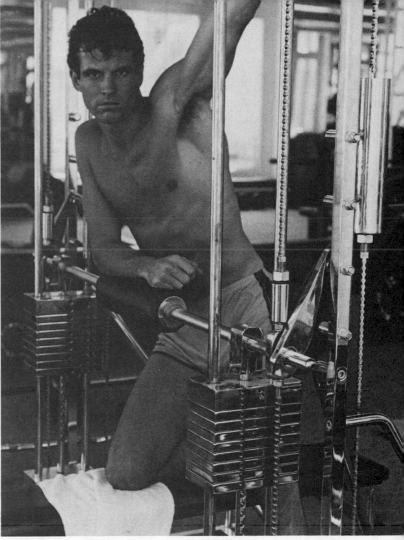

but who want the results that brings. In truth, Nautilus and Universal equipment yield "generalized" development, while more specifically subtle muscular definition is achieved by sophisticated weight-lifting techniques. These nuances are insignificant to the average fellow who is interested only in overall physical enhancement.

Although both Nautilus and Universal machines are excellent, instructions on their use are not included in this book. As with any proprietary equipment, on-the-spot training is highly advisable. Also, such apparatus is so prohibitively expensive that few men can afford it for private use. The aim of this book is to offer only exercises that can readily be performed in the widest possible range of settings, whether in a home, in a backyard, at the beach, or at a gym.

Should you decide either the Nautilus or the Universal approach is the one for you, rush right out and sign up—provided the gym is a first-class joint. If you want to expand your workout to include other types of muscle-building activity, the information will be ready and waiting for you in Chapter 7.

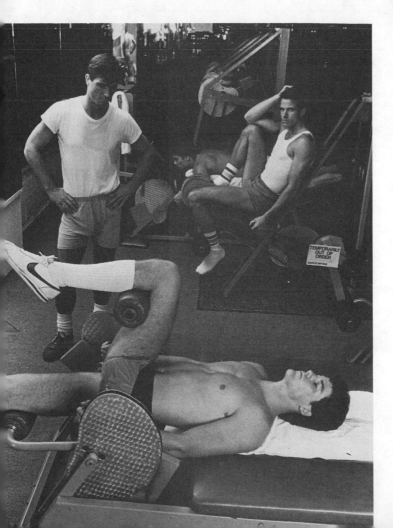

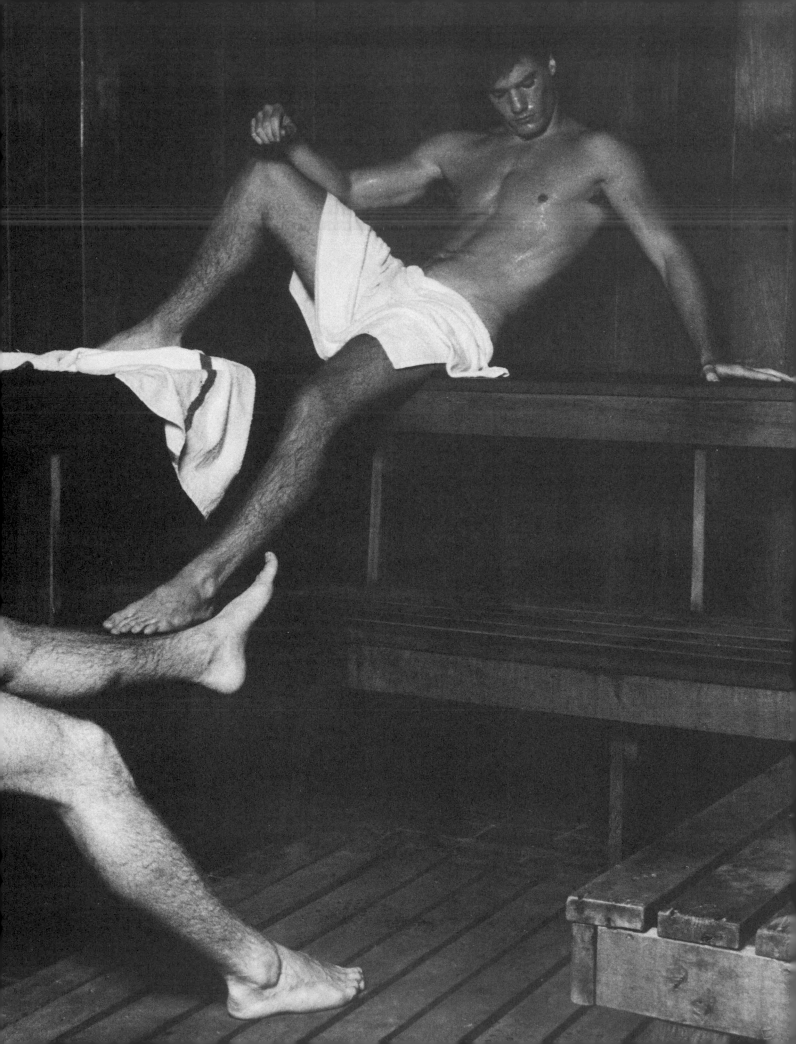

STEAM BATHS

It's commonly believed that all your body's cares drip away in the heated environment of a steam room. A pleasant notion, but not a valid one. What really drips is sweat.

There's nothing wrong with sweating. In fact, if you couldn't perspire, you'd be defunct. But when you sweat too much, you become dehydrated. If you've exercised rigorously, odds are you have already perspired more than your usual share. So why would you consider ending a workout with a trip to a steam room? Because it feels good.

Actually, although steam is pleasure-producing, it never makes sense to hop into a steam room immediately after exercising. Remember, you must always cool down your body upon completing a workout to keep blood from "pooling." And if you don't cool down before the steam treatment, insufficient blood may circulate to the brain, causing you to faint. Even with a decent cooling-off period, it's not unusual for beginners to feel dizzy if they spend more than several minutes in a steam room. Even if you're a steam pro, you can still become drowsy when you bask in it too long.

It's tempting to sit like a lump in a steam bath. That's okay, but it's also a good place to massage your worked body.

Some hardy souls like to plunge into a cold shower straight from the steam room. If your heart is healthy, there's probably no great risk in following their example. It's less startling to your system if you begin showering with warm water and gradually turn it cooler. Why shock yourself?

GYM DANDY

After deciding to join a particular type of gym or club, you still have to settle on the right one for you.

Start out by asking acquaintances if they're gym members. Discuss their likes and dislikes about facilities. Listen most carefully to friends whose temperaments are similar to your own.

If personal endorsements fail to offer any direction, flip through the Yellow Pages. Check off all gyms and clubs convenient to you, then drop by for a firsthand inspection *at the same hour* you plan to do your exercising.

Mentally tune out as your guide sings the establishment's praises. Like used-car salespeople, gym personnel have their selling spiels down pat. They will wax enthusiastic about the benefits of exercise, which you already know. They can be chummy, charming . . . and devious. Never sign a contract on your first visit, even though you can legally cancel within a limited time period (generally three days). As strange as it sounds, enrolling in a gym is akin to purchasing a second home. After all, for the fee you are buying a right of occupancy. You'll be spending part of your life there, at least three times a week. Seemingly minor shortcomings become magnified into serious drawbacks the longer you "inhabit" a gym.

First, size up the gym members on the scene. Are they quiet, congenial, or boisterous? Are they working steadily or chatting in groups? Don't be afraid

SAUNAS

Some gyms promote their sybaritic niceties more than their equipment, and for good reason: Since many fellows regard exercise as drudgery, these guys want to reward themselves after the workout with feel-good extras. That's precisely what a trip to a sauna is—a feel-good extra which has nothing to do with working yourself into shape. But man does not live by exercise alone.

Saunas and steam baths operate on much the same principle, except that saunas employ dry heat and steam baths wet. Also, saunas tend to be much hotter—by as much as 50 to 100 degrees Fahrenheit hotter—so you should be more discriminating in their use. As with steam baths, their appeal is pleasant relaxation. Whether they offer anything else is questionable. Since muscles aren't manipulated, saunas don't tone or enlarge them.

Saunas are hazard-free if you're physically fit— provided you don't camp out in them for more than a quarter-hour—but they're not recommended for anyone in substandard health. The high heat in saunas (and steam baths, too) can prompt vessels to dilate, rushing blood away from the heart to the skin's surface, which in turn causes a drop in blood pressure. The heart tries to reassert normality, and the pulse rate jumps. Obviously, this doesn't bode well for a fellow whose cardiovascular system isn't up to par, but even fit males may feel tired from the strain of a lengthy sojourn in a sauna. Moderation may be boring at times, but it's usually the wisest course.

The weight loss following a sauna treatment is only temporary, the result of prolonged sweating. As soon as you quench your thirst, your body starts retaining fluids again, and you "gain" back what you "lost." Fluid reduction isn't true weight loss.

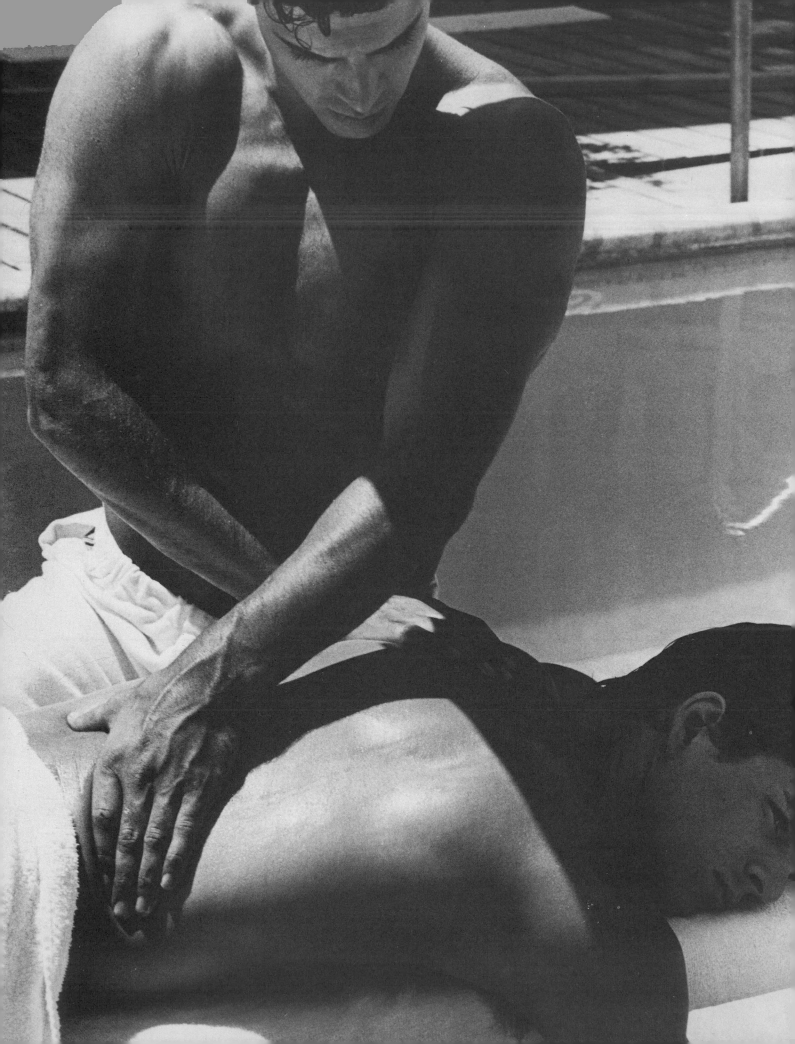

MASSAGE

Massage is therapeutic if you're injured while working out, but it offers much more than therapy.

In truth, massage is not a necessity. But it sure feels good, especially when you're the passive recipient.

Ostensibly, the goal of massage is to reduce tension. Although exercise is inherently relaxing, massage following exercise is advantageous. Waste products build up during exertion, and these must be released to lessen soreness. Kneading movements increase blood circulation, speeding the elimination of wastes.

Experienced masseurs and masseuses can do wonders, but no special training is needed to give a good massage. When no one else is available or will take on the job, you can massage yourself. Just press your fingertips anywhere on your body and start gently rotating. You can stroke, rub, tap, push, vibrate—you can do anything as long as you're not too rough on yourself and it feels good. The warmth from your fingers and hands will warm and soothe whatever area you're working on.

Massage does nothing for the cardiovascular system. It tones muscles but doesn't build them. Who's complaining?

to be a snob: Are they your type of people? Gyms reflect the character of their clientele. Do you want to associate with these people or don't you?

If you don't feel sympathetic with the other members, investigate no further. If they pass inspection, next check out the aesthetics of the place. Is it clean? well lighted? cheery? spacious? inviting? Award-winning decor isn't essential, but if the joint is depressing, forget it—unless you don't care a fig about appearances.

After gauging your general impression of the members and the place, study the equipment. Does it appear to be new and in good repair? Even more important, how much of it is there? Is it all in use? Are members queued up because there's not enough to go around? How long are the lines? If your time is limited—and whose isn't?—a shortage of equipment spells long delays.

If the equipment is sufficient, inquire about the instructors. Is there more than one? At all times? How long have the instructors worked there? Ask

to have them pointed out. Are they seriously instructing or do they appear lackadaisical? It's no good if they're leafing through magazines or telling riotous jokes.

What about the amenities? Is the shower pristine or decrepit? Is there a masseur or masseuse on staff? Is there a pool? whirlpool? sauna? These aren't particularly important to the success or failure of your workouts, but they can make the gym more enjoyable.

Assuming you haven't already rejected the establishment, look closer. How many different types of exercise devices are there? Are they labeled to tell you how they're to be used and for what purpose? (Many gyms don't label equipment; but labels are helpful when you're a novice.) Are there lots of mirrors? (Exercise form is improved when you can watch what you're doing, correcting performance flaws.) Is there a rest area in which to recompose yourself between sets?

Only if you're satisfied on all these counts should you discuss membership. Even if you think the gym is tops, it can't hurt to look into another establishment to compare facilities and fees.

HOME GROWN

If it's financially feasible, gym members should also have some exercise equipment at home. Although this may seem a needless expense, times will arise when at-home workouts will be more convenient than trekking to the gym. It cannot be repeated often enough: Regularity, and regularity alone, gets results. At-home gear helps ensure conscientious commitment.

For an individual who chooses to avoid the gym scene, his own equipment is not an option but a necessity.

Actually, surprisingly little equipment is required to work out at home, since most of the routines outlined in this book don't demand any. But, as you know, to build muscle mass, you must eventually turn to external aids. (As you also know, if you have no intention of increasing the size of your muscles, you won't need any weight-lifting equipment. However, it is almost inconceivable that you would choose to embark on a program to improve your physical fitness and appearance without wanting to augment your muscularity to some degree.)

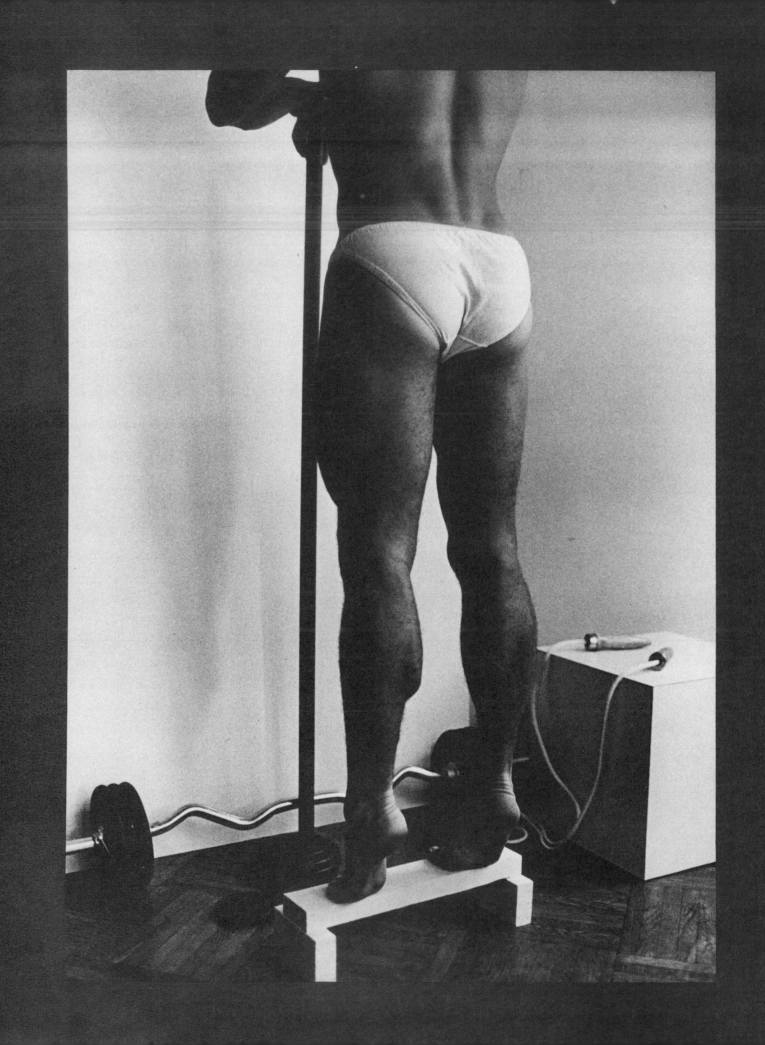

ADEQUATE EQUIPMENT

FULL-LENGTH MIRROR. When you're working out solo with no instructor to supervise you, you are responsible for keeping an eye on your performance. A full-length mirror is invaluable.

MAT. If you have lushly plush wall-to-wall, you may not need an exercise mat. To avoid bruises and injury, you must cushion your body (especially your spine) against hard floor surfaces when you're doing many limbering exercises. An exercise mat is cheaper than a chiropractor.

POLE. If aesthetics don't concern you, you can get by with a broomstick. For certain exercises, you need a rigid pole of some sort to hold on to. (The bar of a barbell, if you have one, also does the trick.)

BOXES. But not the cardboard kind. Three 18-by-18-inch stable wood boxes—sturdy enough to support your weight—are useful in some maintenance and building movements.

(It is possible to improvise, using chairs instead of the boxes, but doing so isn't recommended unless the chairs are very sturdy and unshakable. If the chairs should topple, you might be injured. It's better to search out the cubes in a furniture store, or to make them yourself. When not used for exercising, the cubes can do double duty as end or occasional tables.)

CALF BLOCK. This do-it-yourself project is about the only satisfactory way to work your calves. You need to fasten two 8-inch (give or take a fraction) pieces of two-by-four lumber to about an 18-inch length of two-by-four to create a block you can balance your heels or toes on. (The 8-inchers form the base and rest lengthwise on the floor. See photograph.)

JUMPING ROPE. It's a real aid to aerobic fitness, and is easily stashed in luggage when you're on the road.

DUMBBELLS. You really should invest in weights. If you refuse to purchase an entire system, at least consider dumbbells. They are one-hand-holdable short bars on which you place weight plates at each end. Don't get solid dumbbells, because they don't accommodate interchangeable plates and you would need dumbbells of many different weights to meet the requirements of progressive resistance. As you proceed, the lighter dumbbells become useless. Ideally, the weight plates should include 2 ½-pound plates.

PREFERRED EQUIPMENT

In addition to the equipment listed above, think about obtaining the following for a more efficient workout.

EXERCISE BENCH. For many exercises, it's easier if you have a bench—padded for comfort—to recline on or straddle.

ANKLE WEIGHTS. Naturally, these are weights to wear around your ankles. By making it more difficult to lift your feet, you work out leg muscles more arduously.

BARBELLS. Whereas you need two dumbbells—one for each hand—to work out both arms, you need only one barbell, since barbells have longer poles and are meant to be lifted with both hands. Barbells, which should also have interchangeable weight plates, supplement dumbbells.

LUXURY EQUIPMENT

BENCH WITH RACK. Yup, this is an exercise bench with a rack attachment so you can do bench presses. Some also have attachments for the legs as well, so you can do leg curls. (If you don't know what a bench press or a leg curl is, don't worry about it. By the time you have gone through the whole book, you'll know enough about them to satisfy your curiosity. Neither is a specified exercise in this book because this expensive luxury equipment is needed to perform them.)

EXERCISE BICYCLE. This book doesn't admonish you to pedal an ever-stationary bike because the apparatus is too costly to be considered anything other than a luxury. If you're rolling in dollars, you could make a worse investment. Aerobic benefit is high, and some exercise bicycles come equipped with resistance capabilities.

ROWING MACHINE. Ditto.

TREADMILL. You can run in place without resorting to a treadmill, of course, even without leaving your living room. If you think your exercise-room decor is lacking without a treadmill, spring for one.

QUADRAPHONIC TAPE DECK. Exercising to great music is a great lift.

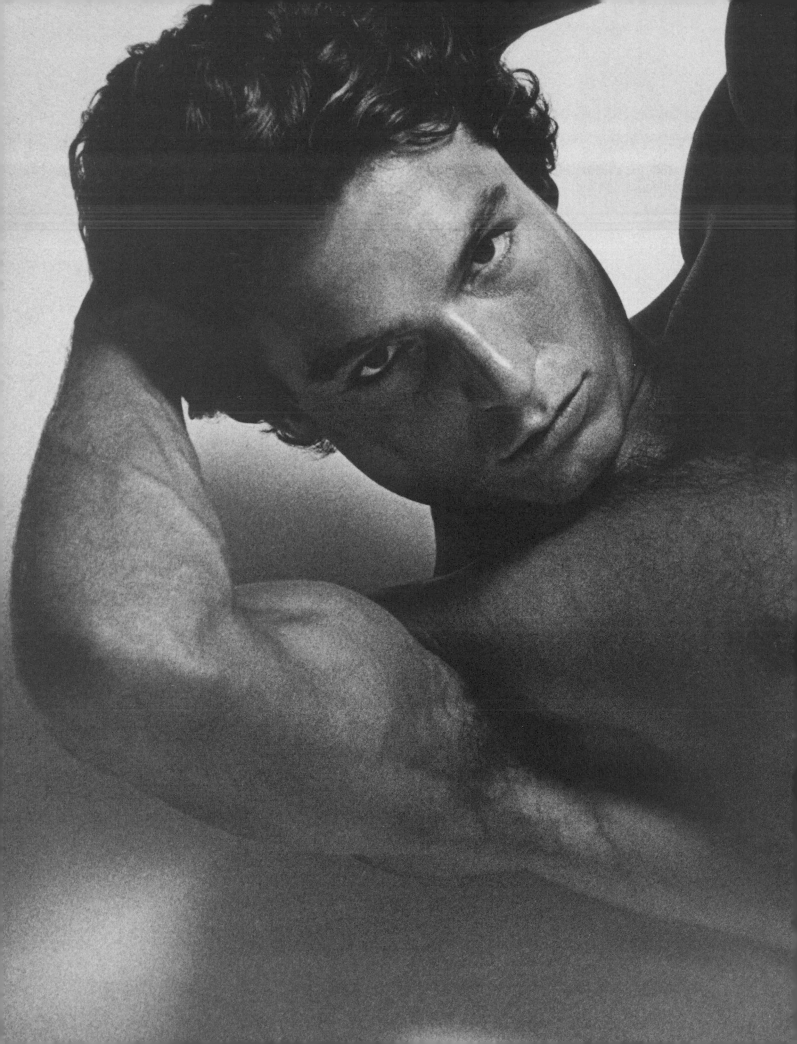

PART II
BODY WORKS

CHAPTER 4

TIME MACHINE

SMART GUY

You already know that a sane warm-up and a sensible cool-down are essential, but just to drive the message home harder, repeat five times: Fools rush in, whereas wise men shape up faster; haste makes wasteful injury.

(A reminder: Since you'll be working out daily, naturally you'll tune up every day. Your warm-up will always be followed by a daily limbering session. When you've completed your stretching routine, you'll move on to the maintenance phase one day, the resistance phase the next day, alternating the two types of exercises on alternate days. Then, each day, you'll conclude the workout with cool-downs.)

Your goal while tuning up is to gently increase your circulation. Unless you're plotting a very specialized exercise program, the order in which you perform your warm-ups truthfully doesn't make a great deal of difference in raising your internal temperature. After all, *all* of you must be prepared. However, there can be a psychological advantage to warming up in a systematic fashion. Most tuning exercises are designed to eliminate mental as well as physical tension. By repeating the same movements in the same sequence every day, you are silently and subconsciously alerting yourself for the rigors ahead while coming to feel more at ease with your body.

Not all the recommended warm-ups are easy stuff. If you're just beginning to work out, you should periodically check your pulse even while tuning up. (And you should never approach your maximum heartbeat at this stage. If you do, you're rushing recklessly . . . or you're in worse shape than you thought. Conversely, if your heartbeat rises only imperceptibly, congratulations.) Nor should you push your body too far too fast past its present flexibility. When an exercise tells you to contort yourself into a configuration your body can't accomplish, simply go through the movements up to the point you can reach without undue strain, then stop.

As you're starting out, read the exercises several times, mentally rehearsing them. Next, with the book in your line of vision, slowly practice the movements without any attempt at perfect execution. Get a sense of the routines by doing them very easily and roughly. Once you've got a generalized feel for the warm-ups, then do them one by one at a snail's pace. (You should follow this procedure when introducing yourself to all the exercises in this book.) Use whatever props appeal to you to catch the spirit. Standing before a full-length mirror helps. If you like classical music, listen to it. If you're more into country, let it twang. Or, if you

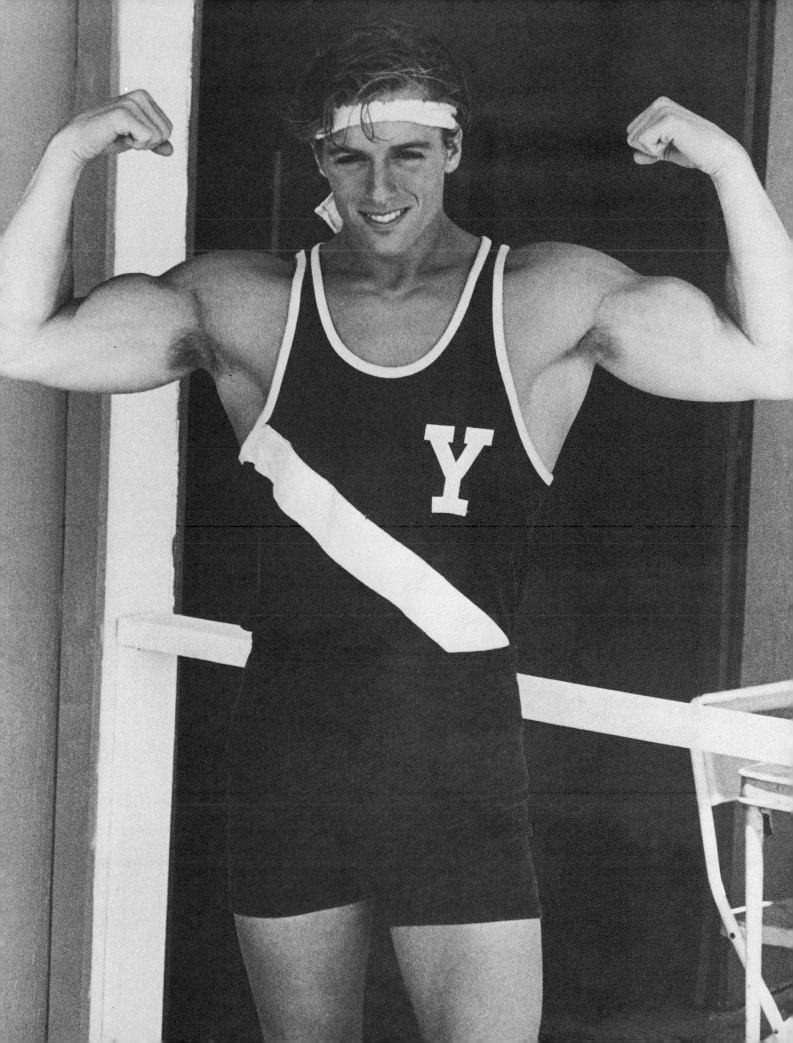

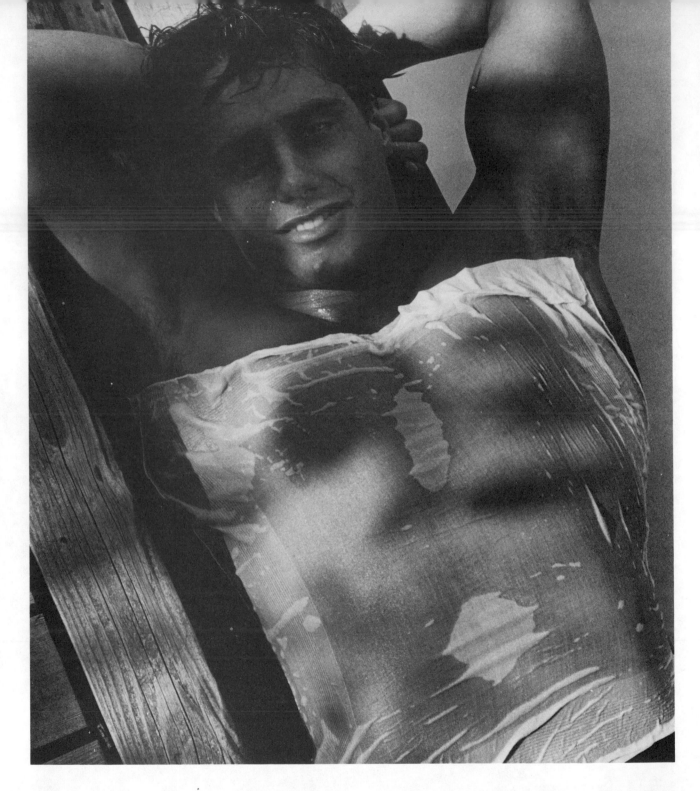

prefer, count—or chant—your own rhythms. Whatever works for you is right.

The number of exercises here and elsewhere is purposely kept minimal so you won't be forced into learning myriad movements. Simplicity is the key to the whole program. From a few exercises large results are attainable.

Even if you're a first-time exerciser, you will be prepared for a safe and thorough workout if you perform all the specified movements at least a couple of times within eight to ten minutes. While you never want to rush, after a while you'll be able to accelerate the pace of the warm-ups somewhat, doing more of them during the same time period, eventually achieving five repetitions. All these variables will be discussed in Chapter 8. Meanwhile, go through the warm-ups as presented, very slowly. Should you choose to adapt the specifics of the warm-up later on, you'll have memorized each step of each exercise by then. And you'll be in far better shape to enjoy your improvisations. After mastering the basics comes the real exhilaration.

THE NECK STRETCH

Since you get the most out of working out when you're free of tension, it's logical to start by tuning up your neck muscles, since emotional uptightness concentrates there, presenting an obstacle to relaxed movement. Breathe deeply throughout the exercise.

Although it is not imperative, you can pull in your abdomen and tighten your buttocks as you go through these movements. Doing so won't warm up the neck any faster, but firming of abdominal and buttocks muscles will occur as a bonus.

Position.

The position of your body is relatively unimportant. You can stand or sit, as long as you keep your back erect with your arms comfortably at your sides.

Progression.

Keeping your chin level, slowly turn your head to the right so that your chin is above your shoulder.

Still keeping a level chin, swivel your head slowly to the left until your chin is above that shoulder.

With chin level and head erect, move your head slowly back and forth, left to right, right to left, progressively stretching farther.

For the second part of this exercise, drop your chin until it nearly touches your chest, then rotate your head slowly and steadily in a continuous circle. As the top of your head dips toward your right shoulder, you will feel the strain on the left side of your neck.

Lifting your chin so that you try to nestle the back of your head between your shoulder blades, continue your rhythmic rotation. You will now feel greater strain on the front neck muscles.

Dipping your head toward your left shoulder, you will experience greater pull on the right side of your neck.

Completing the rotation, as you sweep your chin forward to your chest, the muscles in the back of your neck will be most affected.

Continue rolling your head, slightly increasing the speed and your extension.

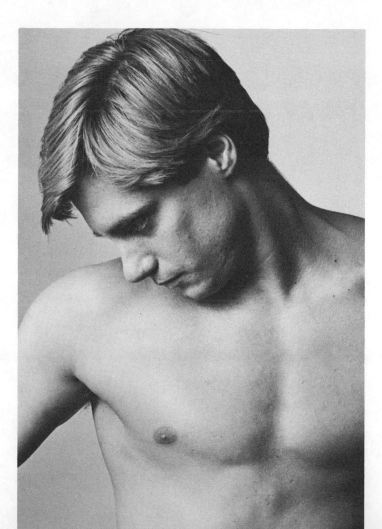

THE SHOULDER SHRUG

Although tension principally manifests itself in the neck muscles, the nearby shoulder muscles are also a tension depository. That's why moving on next to shoulder muscles makes sense. As you tune up here, you will also continue the slow increase of your pulse rate, further warming up your system. Some toning of your upper back muscles also occurs.

Position.

Stand with your feet moderately spread—about eighteen inches to two feet apart—with your arms hanging loosely at your sides, shoulders relaxed.

Progression.

Lift both shoulders simultaneously into a tight shrug, as if you're trying to squeeze them from both sides against your neck.

Hold your shoulders in the raised position for three or four seconds.

Suddenly relax all strain in your shoulder muscles, allowing your arms to drop.

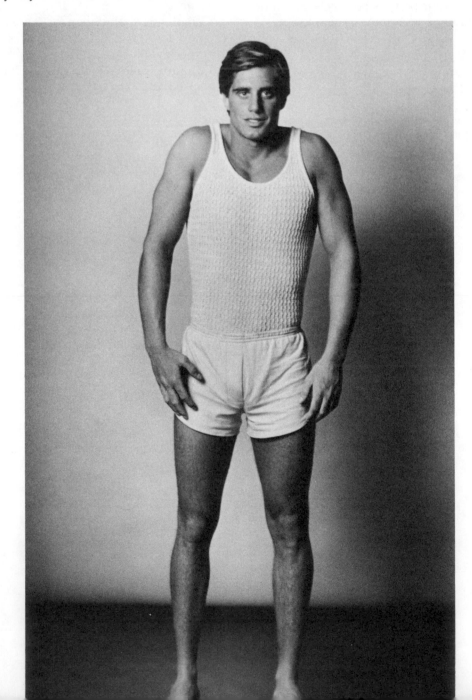

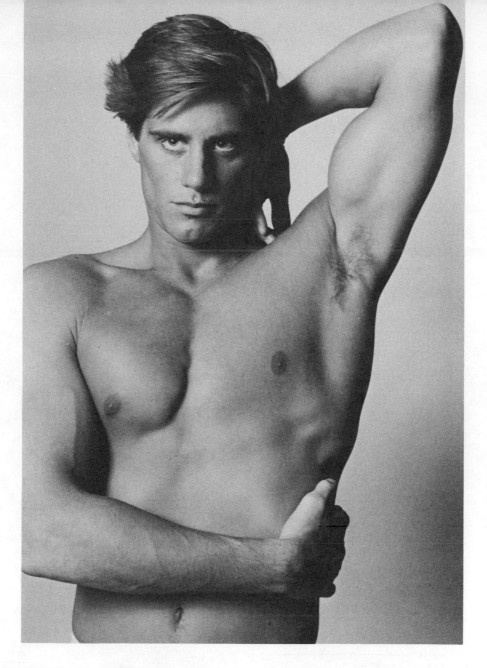

THE "ELBOW-IN-THE-EAR"

Tension can also knot back muscles; to unknot them and to ensure that your workout is not stressful, it's wise to step up your emphasis on shoulder and back muscles now. The following routine is somewhat harder than The Shoulder Shrug, so the gradual increase of your circulation is accelerated in the process. As you're warming up in this exercise, you're also helping to smooth out "love handles" at your waistline.

Position.

A precise starting position isn't crucial. The exercise is easier to complete, however, if you stand with feet slightly spread. With your elbow raised and pointed upward, rest the fingertips of your left hand loosely atop your left shoulder. Crossing your other arm across your torso, clasp your left side with your right hand.

Progression.

Raise your bent elbow as high as possible, as if you were attempting to twist your elbow into your ear.

Relax your muscles and return to the starting position, reversing your movements at a moderate pace.

Do the same with your right elbow.

Alternate between left and right elbow stretches.

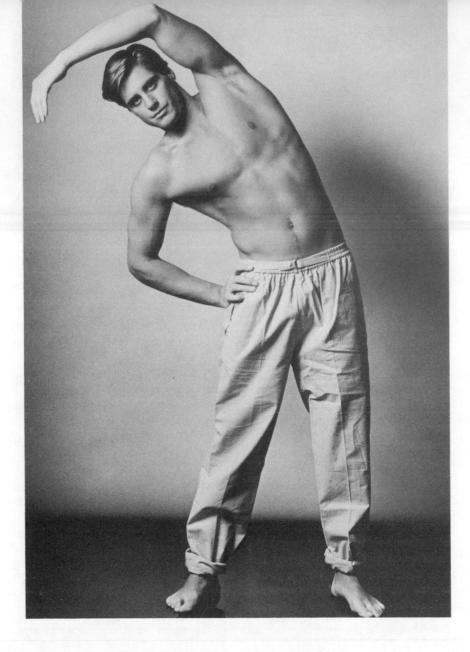

THE BOUNCING BEND

Progressing downward to involve more of your body, you should lift your pace a little. *Gentle* bobbing movements performed rhythmically while you breathe deeply give you a physical and mental lift.

Because you're using more muscles here than in The Elbow-in-the-Ear, your internal body temperature and circulation will continue to climb gradually. At the same time, you're also working out your lower torso, waist, and particularly love handles.

Position.

Stand with your feet slightly spread, your right hand on your hip, your left arm raised in an arc over your head.

Progression.

Bouncing your body only a little to give you momentum, reach with your curved arm past your right shoulder while also lowering your torso sideways to the right, dropping your right shoulder as you go. Keep your hips and legs as stationary as possible, and don't arch your back.

After bouncing/bending as far as possible to the right, slowly bounce back to your original position.

Change hands, placing your left hand on your left hip and raising your right arm in an arc over your head.

Bounce and bend as far as possible to the left.

Alternate between your left and right sides.

THE FORWARD FLOP

Until now, you've been concentrating primarily on the upper half of your body. Time to bring your lower half slowly into focus. Whenever you bend at the waist, lowering your torso closer to the ground while keeping your feet flat on the floor, you work out a whole series of muscles while also bringing leg muscles (particularly your "hamstrings," the muscles backing up your thighs) more actively into play. Should you have any residual tension—although you shouldn't—extra bobbing completes your relaxation. Naturally, this flopping augments blood flow throughout your body and progressively warms muscles.

Position.

Stand straight with legs slightly spread and arms hanging loosely at your sides.

Progression.

Slowly allow your body to flop loosely forward, keeping your arms parallel with your unbending legs.

Gently bounce your torso, taking your head closer to your knees and your hands closer to the floor.

While you continue the slow bouncing movements, move to an upright position again.

Without pausing, begin your casual forward flop again, extending progressively farther downward.

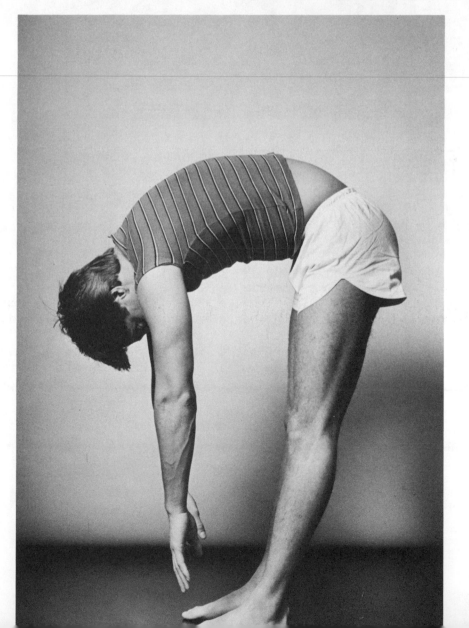

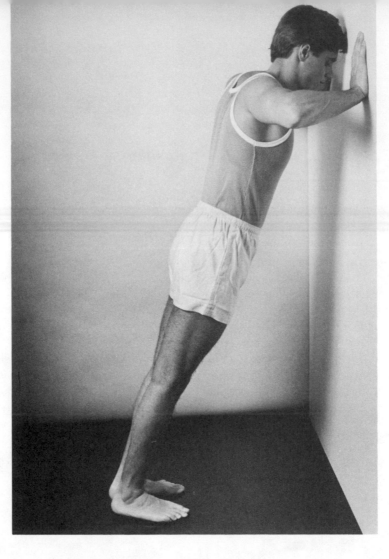

THE OFF-THE-WALL

This exercise works out several areas while generally warming you up, but its major contribution is protecting the Achilles tendon, that area behind your ankle which is so subject to injury, particularly as a result of running. Tendinitis—inflammation of the tendon—is caused by strain on the muscles surrounding and attached to the tendon. The tighter the muscles, the more likely they'll be strained, and the area can become painfully swollen. The only way you can prepare the Achilles tendon for more rigorous exercise is by stretching nearby muscles carefully before you become too active. Jerky or sudden movements are particularly hard on tendons, so be sure you take this exercise slow and easy. Even when you're treating yourself tenderly, your tune-up will keep going.

Position.

Standing about a yard from a wall with your feet flat on the floor and your body erect, extend your arms to the wall and rest your palms, separated by your shoulder width, against the wall.

Progression.

Slowly bend your elbows—while keeping your feet flat on the floor—until your head almost touches the wall.

Hold this position for seven seconds.

Push against the wall while straightening your elbows until you return to the original position.

THE CHEST/THIGH EMBRACE

This exercise is particularly good for back muscles. Although the relatively easy motions might seem to be a break in the routine, the foot movement contributes significantly to your tune-up. The flexing of the feet helps work out your calf muscles, and calves are among the most difficult areas to shape up. Similarly, the muscles in the feet are not often subjected to a full range of movement, which means they're usually underused. Rotating the feet, causing the ankles to move sideways, reduces the possibility of foot sprains while also increasing coordination. Breathing deeply is extra-important during this one.

Position.

Lie on the floor with your knees bent. Breathe deeply and relax, trying lightly to press your spine as close to the floor as possible.

Progression.

Cup your palms around your knees and pull them toward your chest. Keep your back flat against the floor and don't raise your head.

As you bring your knees forward, wrap your arms across your shins as if you were embracing them.

Hugging your shins more tightly, pull your thighs against your chest until thighs and chest are firmly compressed.

Holding this position, flex your feet so that your toes point toward your chin.

Slowly rotate your feet in a circle, flexing and unflexing your toes.

Slowly lower your feet to the floor until you have returned to the original position.

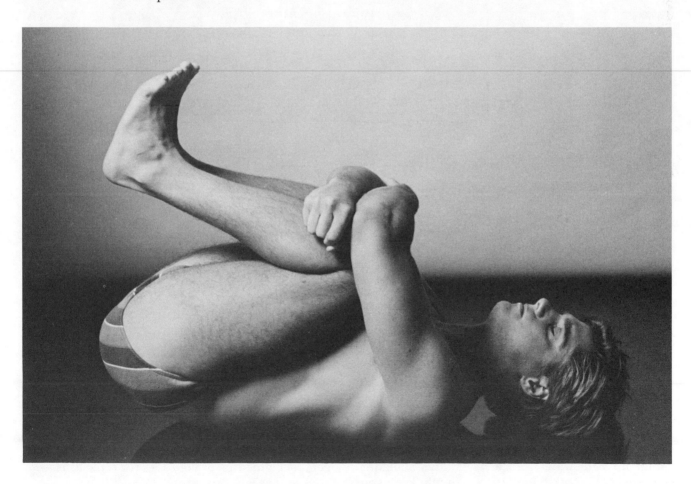

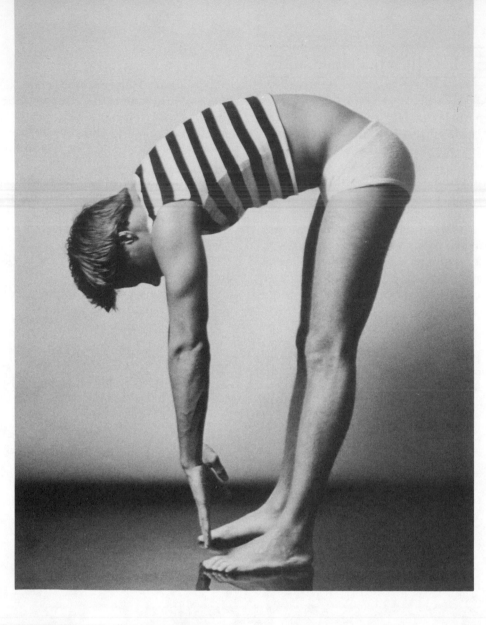

THE TOE TOUCH

Another area especially prone to injury is the hamstrings. That's because of their location behind the usually more massive thighs, causing a muscular imbalance. Whenever one muscle moves in one way, an opposing muscle moves in the other direction. Ideally, these opposing muscles should be equally strong, but in the case of hamstrings and thighs (quadriceps, frequently called quads), this is seldom true. So a vital part of your tune-up is protecting the hamstrings through stretching them, just as a major part of your overall workout is to build up hamstrings. Since hamstrings straighten the knees, to work them out you should keep your knees straight. But straight does not mean taut like the spring of a steel trap. That type of rigidity pro-

motes injury too. Although it sounds contradictory, try to think about straightening your knees to a loose lock.

Position.

With your feet fairly close together—separated by only six inches or so—and your legs straight, keeping your back fairly rigid, bend forward a little from the waist, allowing the force of gravity to keep your hanging arms parallel to your legs.

Progression.

Slowly bend forward, keeping feet flat on the ground and knees braced, until the tips of your fingers touch the tips of your toes (or come as close to your toes as you can reach).

Hold this position for seven seconds.

Raise yourself slowly to the standing position.

THE LUNGE

Now that you're approaching the end of your warm-up, you should move faster to loosen up even more. The jumping that's involved in this exercise helps boost circulation; gets your buttocks, thigh, and hamstring muscles all more actively into the act; and generally helps build your endurance.

Position.

Stand straight with feet fairly close together.

Progression.

Take a slight jump, simultaneously thrusting your right leg forward and pushing your left leg behind, landing on the balls of your feet but immediately thereafter planting your feet flat on the floor. The right (front) leg should be bent; the left (back) one should be reasonably straight. While you are moving your legs in these opposite directions, at the same time raise your left arm straight upward in front of you, angled toward the horizon, while extending your right arm at a downward angle behind you.

Keeping your feet flat, lower your body closer to the floor by bending your bent right knee more. Keep your back straight and your left leg locked at the knee.

Bouncing a bit to push off, jump, reversing your legs and arms so that your right leg moves behind you while your left leg comes forward. Likewise, switch the position of your arms. When you land, your left leg should now be bent in front of you and your right leg should be straight behind you; your right arm should be pointing upward in front of you, your left arm pointing downward behind.

Flat-footed once more, lower yourself closer to the floor by bending your knee.

Repeat, increasing your stretches and bends.

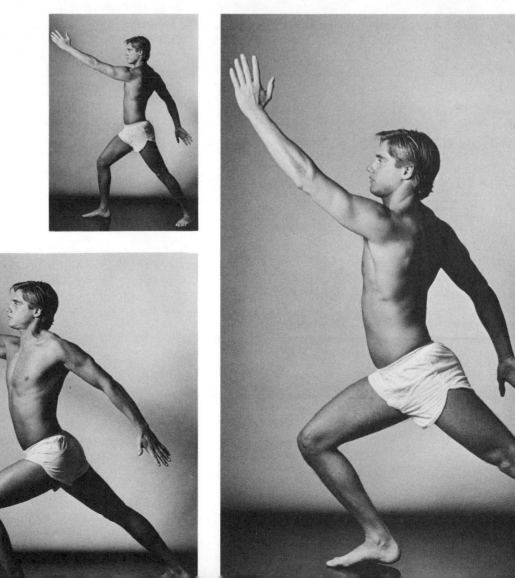

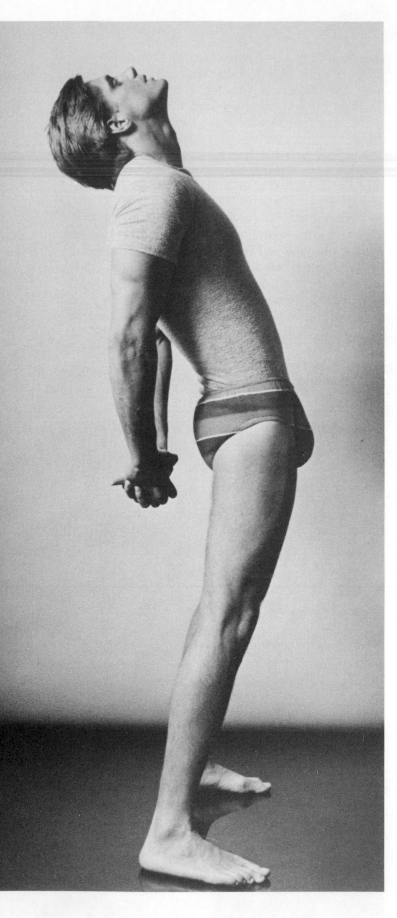

THE STRADDLE STRETCH

Here is another exercise that stimulates circulation throughout your entire body, even though its pace is slower than that of The Lunge. By now, your body should be adequately warmed. This routine is sort of an insurance policy. It works out various muscles, stretching the spine for greater flexibility while firming the buttocks and inner thighs. Because of the full range of movement—and because you'll shortly be moving on to another group of exercises—remember to take it slowly, so you can build up your energy reserve.

Position.

With feet flat on the floor and spread about a foot apart, arms straight and hands clasped together behind your back, bend your body back from the waist.

Progression.

Bending backward from the waist and pushing downward from the shoulders, extend your stretched arms back as if to make a perpendicular angle with the floor.

Slowly bend back even farther and hold the position for three seconds. (Not shown.)

Slowly raise your body upright, lifting your arms at the same time, and bend forward while continuing to lift and rotate the arms until you are bent as far forward as possible and your arms are angled straight up behind your head, pointing to the ceiling.

As the next part of the exercise, unclasp your hands and swing your arms around until they are parallel to your legs.

'Clasp your hands again, in front this time. Bend your knees slightly, and place your clasped hands between your legs until they are behind your knees.

Tense your abdominal muscles; tighten your buttocks. Force your arms back even farther between your legs, keeping your feet flat on the floor. Hold the position for three seconds.

Next, bring your arms back slightly in front of your feet. Drop your palms down to the floor for balance, then slowly spread your feet as wide apart as possible without bending your knees. At your widest extension, hold the position for five seconds.

Slowly bring your feet closer together, then stand and resume the original stance. Repeat the entire routine.

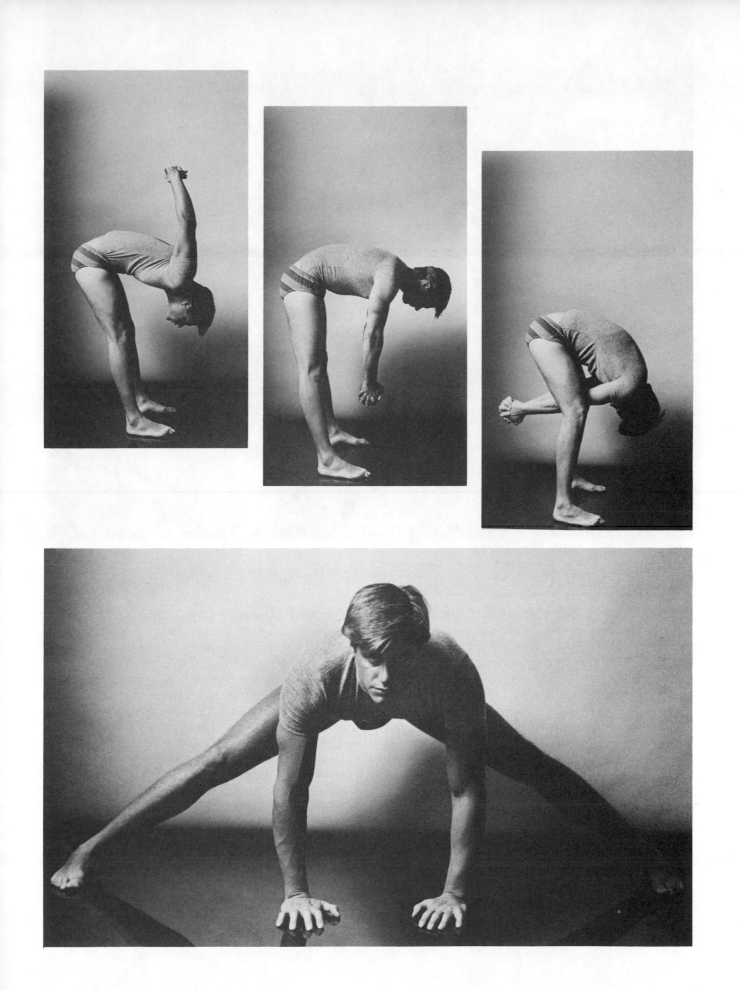

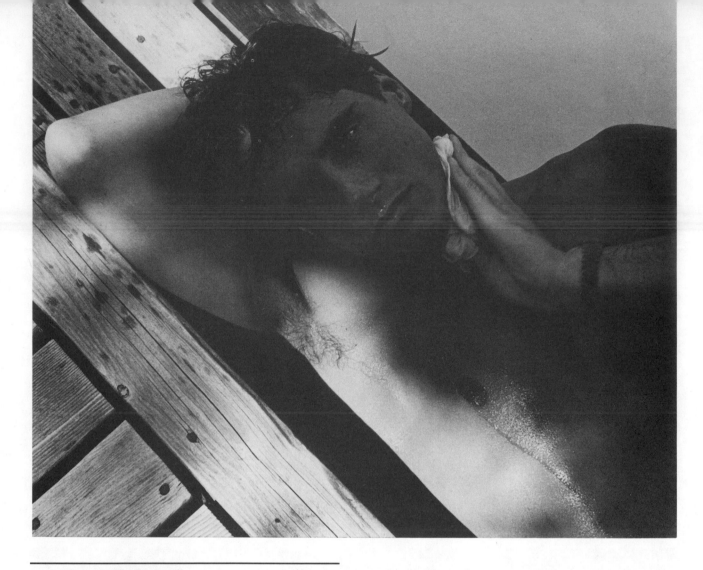

HAPPY ENDING

To avoid backfires after a steady workout, you *must* perform cooling-down exercises. If you're already convinced of this, good. If you're not, don't expect a happy conclusion to the workout. Your muscles will be smarting tomorrow and you'll wish you had been smarter today.

The type of cool-downs you do is less important than making sure you do cool down, allowing your heart to return to a more normal beat. One way is simply to walk slowly, meandering here and there. Although doing so accomplishes that goal, that's all it does accomplish. It's possible to cool down and to get some extra benefit at the same time by slowly stretching your body. A good stretch after a workout also gets rid of carbon dioxide and other wastes accumulated during exercise better than a subdued stroll.

To be honest, the recommended cool-downs call for a certain degree of expertise. The first—or second or third—time out, you may not be able to see these exercises to the described finish. Just go as far as you can without forcing your body, then stop.

As you progress, your flexibility will increase rapidly and dramatically.

The more often you exercise wisely, the sooner your muscles will be primed for more concentrated efforts. This fact is applicable to cool-downs too. Ideally, your body will have been thoroughly warmed during the workout, so your cool-downs, although involving a fair measure of stretching, should be performed without too much strain. On the other hand, if you're exhausted by the time you reach the cool-down stage and are unable to execute the movements completely even after you've been exercising regularly, learn to pace yourself better.

During cool-downs, to get the full benefit, never bobble your body to increase your extension. This will warm you up rather than cool you down. Go through the movements slowly, stretching and holding as indicated. As always, stay attuned to your body.

The whole point of cooling down is to do it gradually. No matter what level of expertise you reach, allow at least five to eight minutes for your cool-down, spending a couple of minutes on each of the following exercises.

THE ANKLE HOLD

Position.

With feet together, back and arms straight, bend forward while keeping your knees locked.

Progression.

Maintaining a rigid back and tight knees, slowly continue bending forward.

Clasp your calves and hold briefly.

Still keeping your back as straight as possible and your knees locked, bend forward farther.

If possible, clasp your ankles.

Hold this position for two or three seconds, sucking in your abdominal muscles and tightening your buttocks.

Release your ankles and slowly resume an upright position.

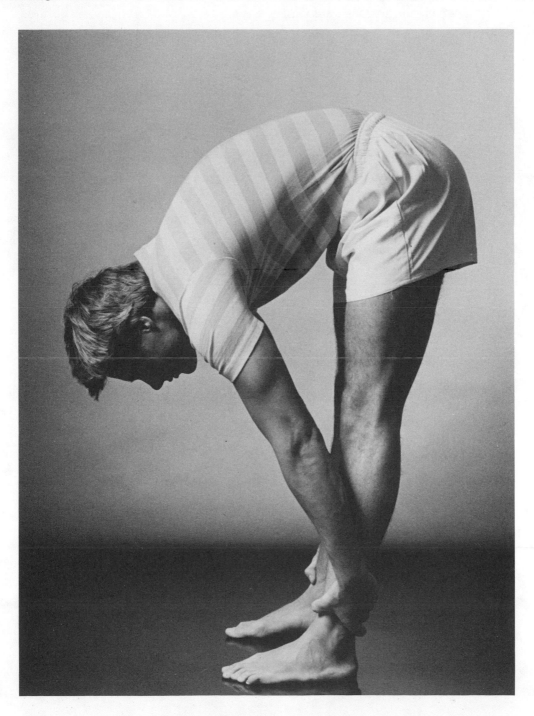

THE SIDE WINDER

Position.

Seated on the floor, stretch your legs their widest without bending them. Raise your arms above your head with your elbows slightly bent.

Progression.

Without rotating your hips, turning only from the chest and shoulders, swivel your torso toward your right thigh.

Bending forward, stretch your arms as if to clasp your right foot.

Lean your whole torso closer to your thigh and keep reaching for your foot, moving beyond it if possible.

Pause. Breathe deeply. Slowly raise yourself to the original position.

Repeat on your other side.

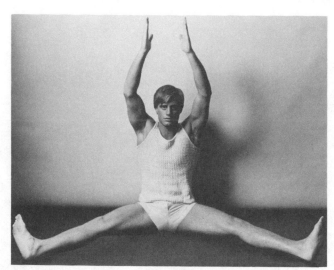

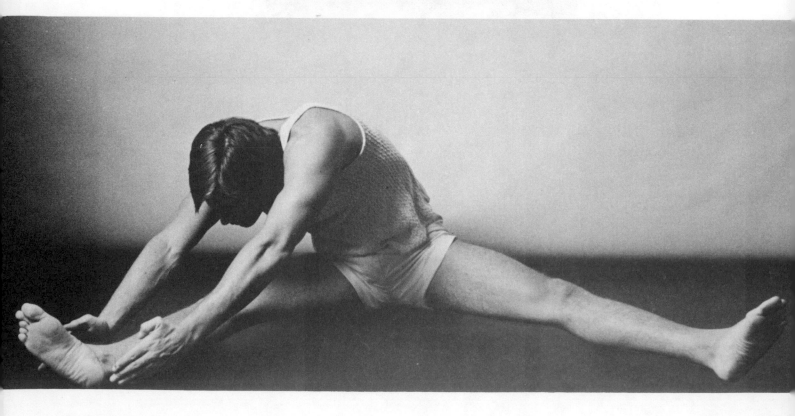

74

THE "PRAISE-THE-HEAVENS"

Position.

Kneeling on the floor with your knees close together, sit with your buttocks on the floor, your feet just slightly wider than your hips.

Progression.

Slowly arch your back backward, using your elbows for support.

Lean back as far as you can to contemplate the heavens (or the ceiling).

Pause, holding the position, sucking in your abdominal muscles and tightening your buttocks.

Slowly raise yourself in fluid, not bouncing, movement.

Repeat, holding longer.

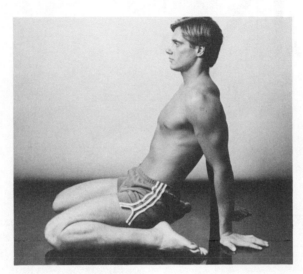

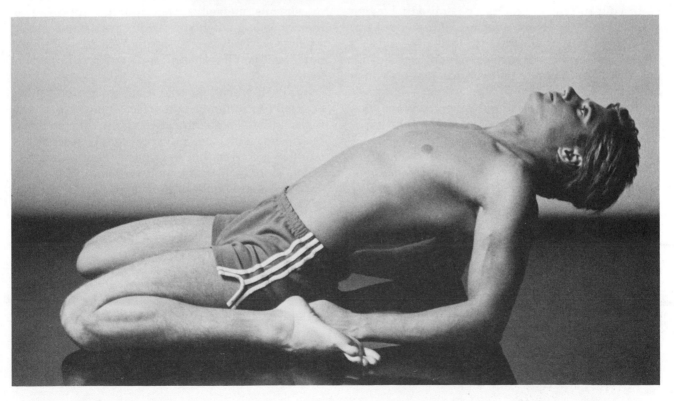

CHAPTER 5

SMOOTH SAILING

EVERY WHICH WAY

Once your internal temperature is raised following a warm-up, your body is primed for stepped-up, injury-free concentration on stretching the muscles for greater flexibility and coordination. Haste is not desirable during the limbering phase—which should be pursued faithfully every day—but good form is. *Feel* your muscle movement. *Picture* what you're doing while you're doing it. Don't be impatient.

In the workout cycle, limbering movements promote body health and awareness by keeping your muscles on guard. Unstretched muscles are lazy muscles that balk when asked to perform a job. Well-stretched muscles are ever ready.

But overstretched muscles are painful. The most common mistake made while limbering is to bounce and jerk the body to achieve greater extension. Such jolts shock the muscles in much the same way as plucking at a taut rubber band. Just as the rubber band can snap, your muscles can tear. Slow, rhythmic stretching is less traumatic and much more effective.

Eventually, rest assured, you will be able to complete all the limbering exercises prescribed . . . but

"eventually" could mean six months or a year down the road. If you try to do them all to the letter right away, you'll probably become sore and sorely discouraged. As previously advised, first rehearse the movements mentally, then roughly approximate them, heeding when your body says "Halt." Later, when your body stops saying "No more," think how great you'll feel. And how much better you'll look.

But even when you take it all faster, don't push yourself to a huff-and-puff stage. The whole reason for sailing into limbering after tuning up is to make certain you don't deplete your energy reserve before moving on to the next phase of your workout. If you shoot your wad here, you'll be unable to get it up again for what's to come later.

You should spend about fifteen to twenty minutes limbering before moving on to either maintenance or building exercises (depending on whether aerobics or progressive resistance is scheduled for that particular day). At this point, you may not be able to do all the specified stretches as described within that time period—you may not be supple enough to do all of them perfectly within *any* time limit right now—without straining yourself unduly; but keep in mind that your long-range goal is to perform each of these exercises five times during your limbering phase. For the moment, depending

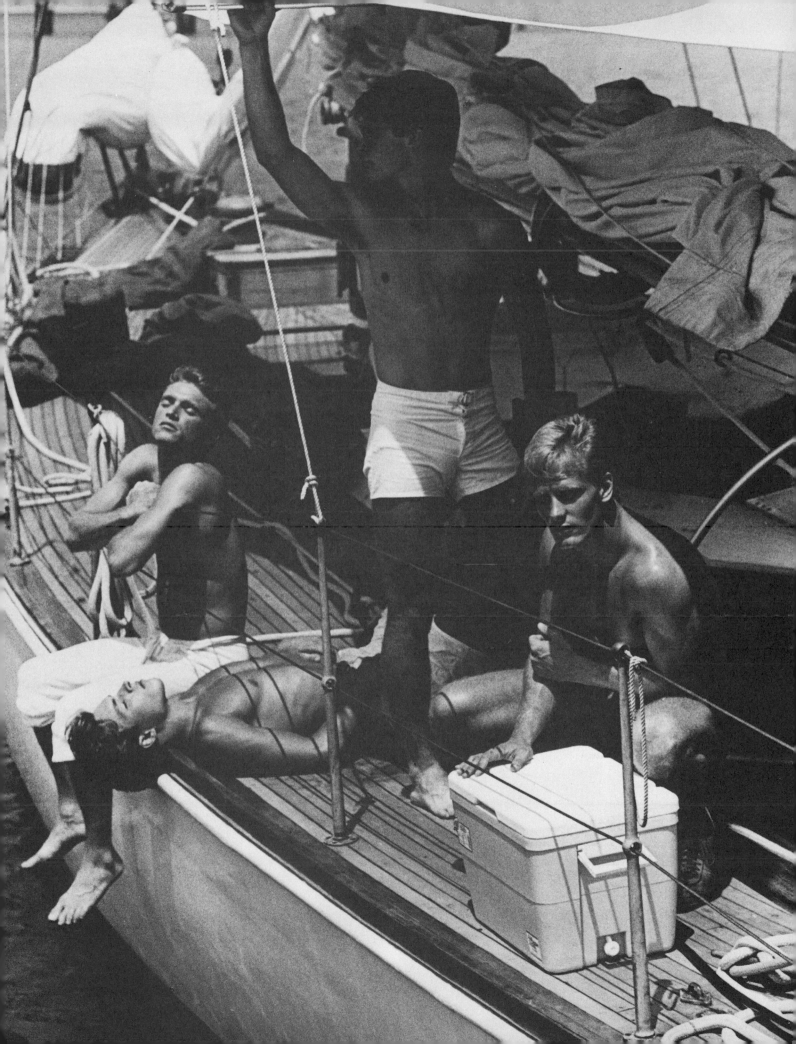

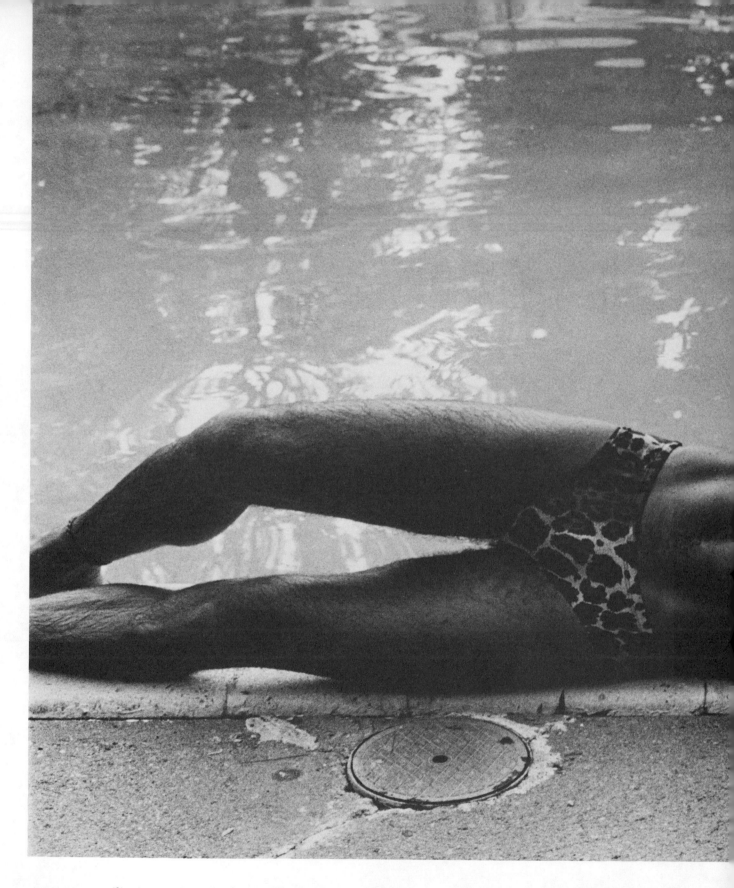

upon your agility, ten minutes of casual limbering might be your limit.

When you're a whiz at these limbering movements, you'll probably choose to concentrate on certain ones over others in keeping with the goals of particular workouts. For now, though, get a feel for all the specified movements. In combination, they stretch your entire body. A well-toned body is the

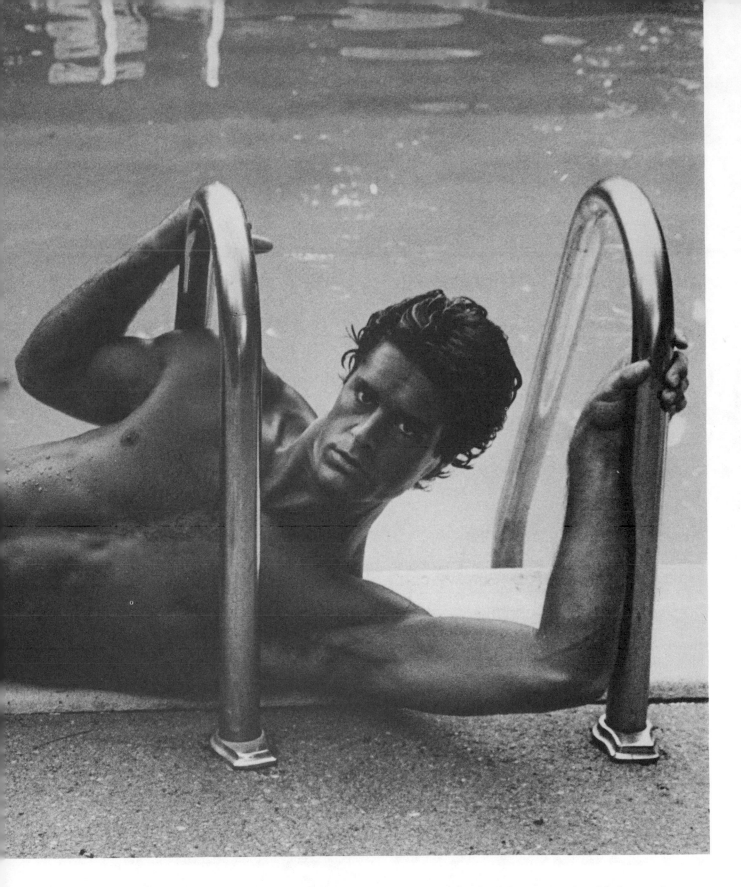

result of a total stretching program. Don't be deceived by the relatively small number of exercises involved. They do a big—and complete—job.

Since your tuning exercises incorporated a fair amount of stretching, you shouldn't require any special preparation before going into limbering. But do remember that deep breathing is always a part of the plan.

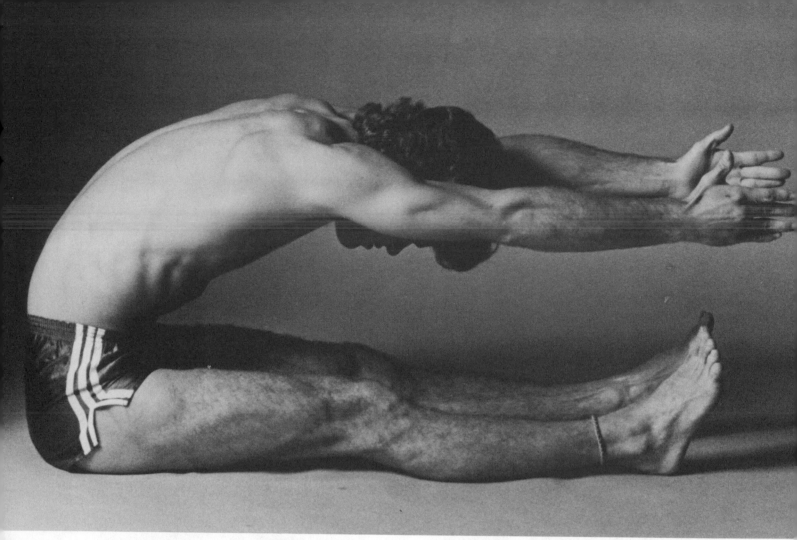

THE SEATED TAKE-A-BOW

This is a good exercise to start with because it ensures that the vulnerable hamstrings are conditioned. You should also feel a contraction of the abdominal muscles, and firming the abdomen is almost every man's goal.

Position.

Sit on the floor (or exercise mat) with your legs fairly close together—your ankles no more than a foot apart—and straight out in front of you.

Progression.

Raise your arms straight above you, palms facing each other at a distance of about a foot. Breathe deeply and reach for the ceiling, with the reach seemingly coming from above your elbows through your forearms rather than from your shoulders, which should not be raised or hunched. Your back should be straight and your chin level. Keep stretching upward.

Sucking in your abdominal muscles, continue your s-m-o-o-t-h upward reach; then slowly bend forward from the waist, keeping your back straight but tucking your chin closer to your chest. Sweep slowly forward as if honoring pagan gods.

Bend until your arms are parallel to your legs. Keep stretching your arms, extending your hands above your toes or beyond them if possible. (Because your arms are parallel with your legs, your hand level will probably be a few inches above the tips of your toes.)

Taking another deep breath, slowly lift your back, arms, and chin to their original position.

THE GRAB-A-BOW

This variation on The Seated Take-a-Bow is more demanding on the hamstrings while helping to stretch your lower back. The exercise is also good for your waist.

Position.

Seated on the floor with your legs straight out in front of you, bring your legs together until your ankles touch.

Progression.

Taking a deep breath, bend forward as in The Seated Take-a-Bow, but don't stop when your arms are parallel to your legs. Instead, keep leaning forward and reaching farther.

If possible, grab your ankles. Otherwise, grab whatever is handy, perhaps your calves. If necessary, bend your knees somewhat, although preferably not.

Flex your feet, pointing them, and especially your toes, toward your lowered head. Your chin should be close to your chest.

As you flex your feet, suck in your abdomen and tighten your buttocks, lifting your feet an inch or two off the floor.

Move your torso as near to your legs as possible.

Hold the position for a few seconds, then slowly resume an upright position, keeping your heels off the floor if possible.

Lift your feet a few inches again before lowering your heels almost to the floor, keeping your butt and gut taut.

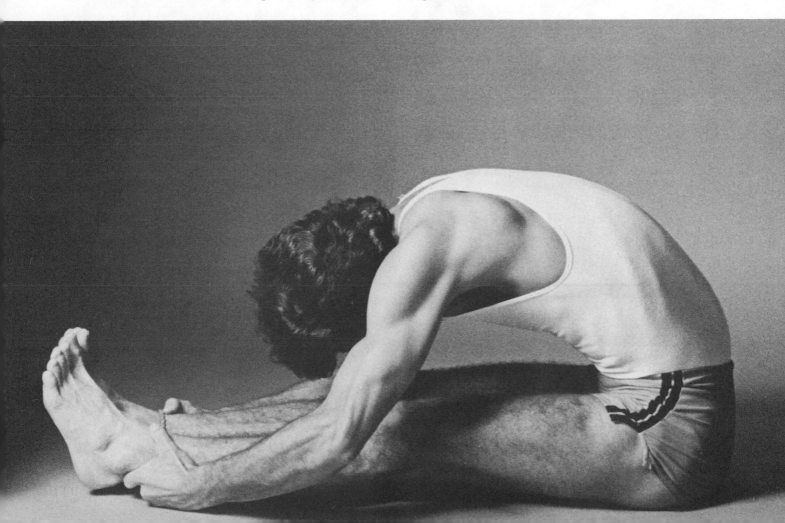

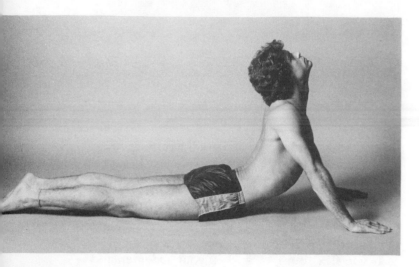

THE UPLIFT

For a change of pace, now you'll go into a different exercise specifically designed to stretch the lower back and also to trim away any softness there. The entire body is worked, however, thereby increasing total flexibility.

Position.

Lie face down with your arms at your sides, elbows bent and palms on the floor beside your chest.

Progression.

Trying *not* to use your hands exclusively for leverage but relying on your back and waist muscles for a good assist, lift yourself up from the waist until your chest and belly are both off the ground and your arms are straight, palms on the floor and elbows stiff.

Arching your back and lifting your chin, gaze at the ceiling for a second or two.

Slowly lower yourself to the original position.

As the next part of the exercise, push your arms straight back beside your body—palms up—and bend your knees until the heels of your flexed feet are as close to the back of your legs as possible.

Clasp your ankles, lift your head, take a deep breath.

Pulling your ankles, arch your back and lift both your legs and your chest. Hold for five seconds.

Slowly lower yourself to the floor again.

Reposition your arms as for the beginning position and go through all the movements again.

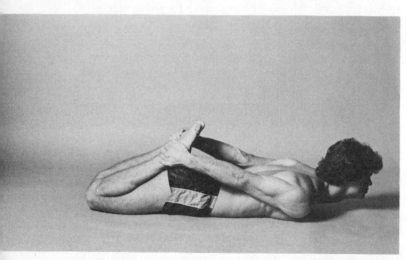

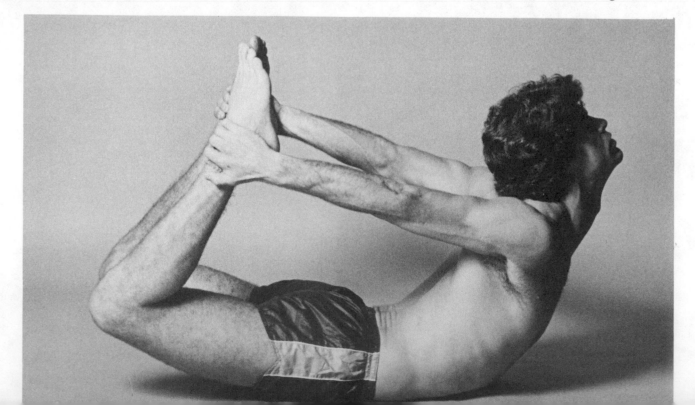

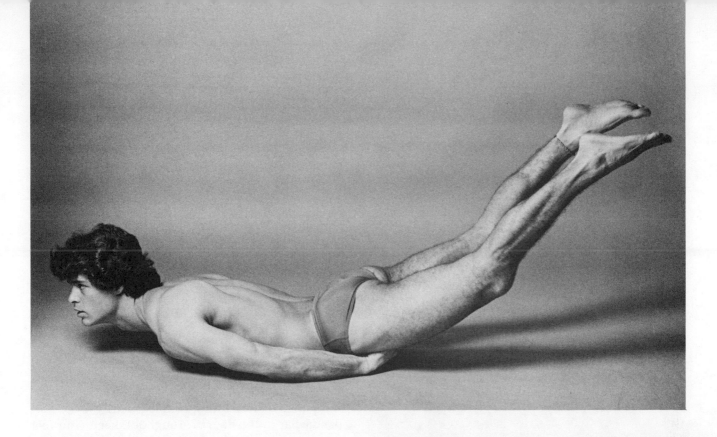

THE CLICK

This one sounds easier than it really is, so if The Click gives you some trouble, don't worry. You'll master it in time. The exercise is particularly good for strengthening and defining the muscles on either side of the spine reaching down the lower back. It's even better for eliminating any droop to the buttocks.

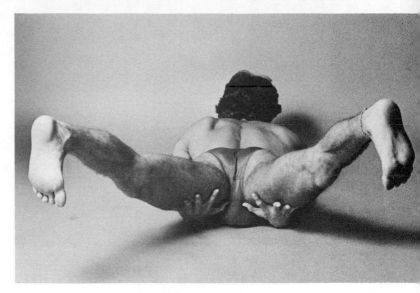

Position.

Lie face down with your arms bent so your palms can be placed comfortably against your pelvis.

Progression.

Arch your neck back so your chin is pointing at an upward angle.

With your feet about a foot apart, lift your legs to at least a 45-degree angle if possible. Don't arch your back for extra leverage. Try to keep your chest flat to the floor.

Taking a deep breath, slowly spread your legs wide without lowering them. Keep your feet flexed and your toes curled.

Exhaling slowly, with your buttocks muscles held tight, bring your legs slowly back together again until your heels "click." Try to keep your legs high and reasonably straight.

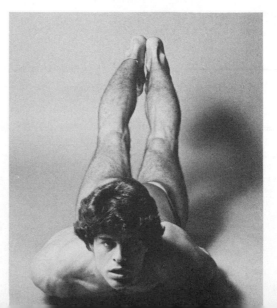

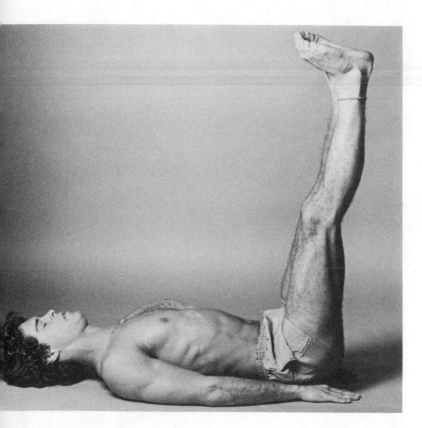

THE CIRCLE

Like The Click, The Circle works out the buttocks muscles, but it puts new emphasis on firming up your inner thighs and flattening your abdomen.

Position.

Lie flat on your back with your arms straight, your hips resting comfortably on top of your hands. Your palms should be flat on the floor.

Progression.

Take a deep breath, suck in your gut, then slowly raise your legs—keeping them straight, no bend at the knees—until they're a few inches off the floor. Release your breath.

If possible, keep lifting your legs until they're perpendicular to the floor. Throughout, keep your feet flexed and your toes curled. You shouldn't arch your back while lifting your legs.

Rotating both legs simultaneously, slowly open them wider, dropping them to complete a lopsided circle, stopping when your ankles come together a few inches off the floor.

Don't rest your feet on the ground. Hold them suspended for a few seconds while tightening both your belly and your buttocks muscles.

Relax your gut and butt.

Draw another deep breath and start over again without ever dropping your feet to the floor.

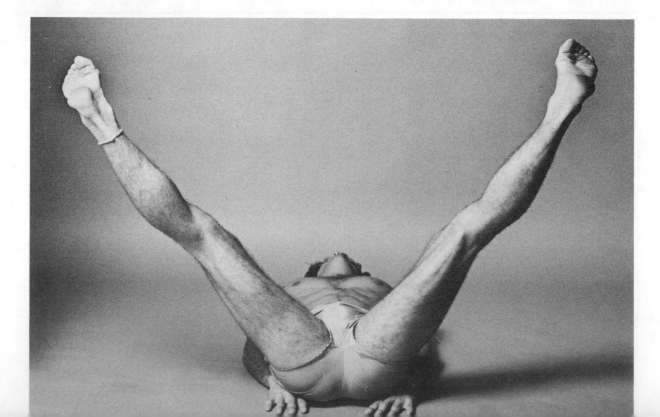

THE LEG-IN

More help for your abdomen. (By the way, any movement that aids the abdomen also helps the lower back.) Also, some particular help for firming up your waistline.

Position.

Lie flat on your back resting your hips on the tops of your hands as in The Circle.

Progression.

Lift your feet—keeping your legs straight and close together, feet flexed—about six inches off the floor.

Tighten your abdominal and buttocks muscles for a few seconds, then relax them slightly.

Bending your knees, slowly bring your thighs as close as possible to your chest. Don't lift or arch your back.

Slowly reverse your movements, stretching your legs straight out without allowing your heels to touch the ground. Stop instead about six inches off the floor.

Tighten your abdominal and buttocks muscles again, and repeat the leg movement without letting your heels touch the floor.

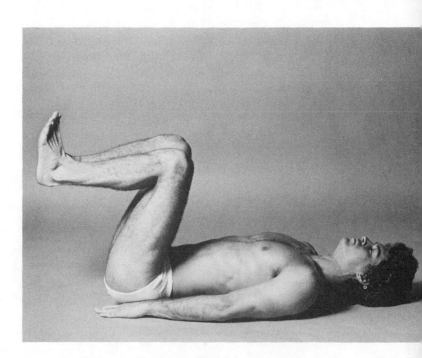

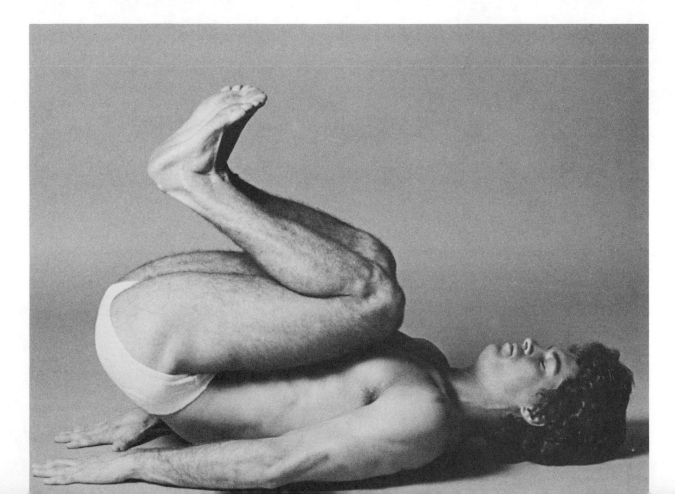

THE ANGLE STRETCH

Not every man has the perseverance to attain a "washboard belly," but working out the abdomen has special priority. There's no way your body can look its best if your abdomen isn't firm and hard. That's why your workout is always strong on abdominal exercises. This one, in addition to benefiting that area, also gets at your shoulders, neck, hamstrings, buttocks, even your groin.

Position.

Lie on the floor, pressing your spine as flat as possible, with your knees bent and your arms beside you.

Progression.

As if you were doing The Chest/Thigh Embrace (page 67), draw your legs up until your chest and thighs are compressed, your feet flexed with your toes pointed toward your chin.

Taking a deep breath and exhaling as you proceed, contract your abdominal muscles as you raise your head and drop your chin while slowly lifting your legs to about a 45-degree angle. As you raise your legs, simultaneously lift your shoulders off the floor and raise your arms until they're straight and parallel to your legs.

Tense your abdomen and buttocks muscles, drawing in your breath.

Lower your shoulders to the floor and bring your thighs back to your chest, pulling against your shins to compress more tightly. Keep your feet flexed.

Lift both arms and legs again to that 45-degree angle without putting your feet on the floor.

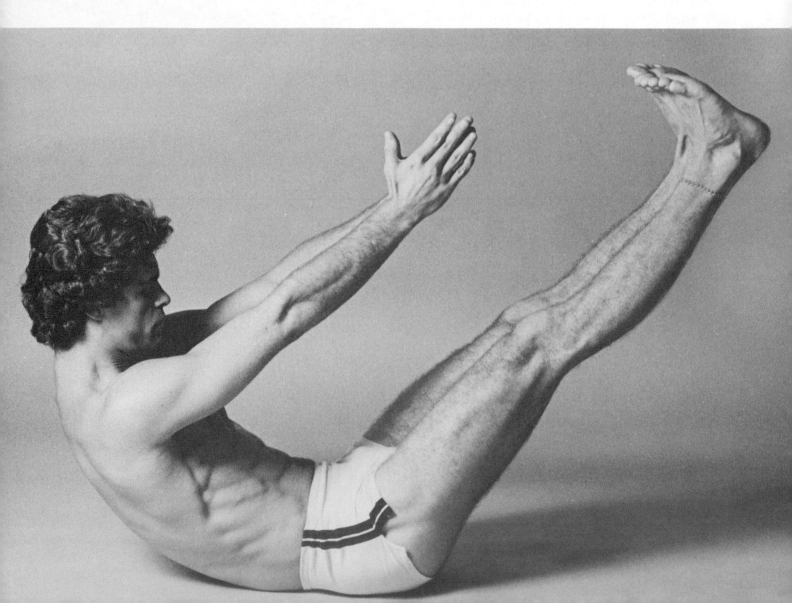

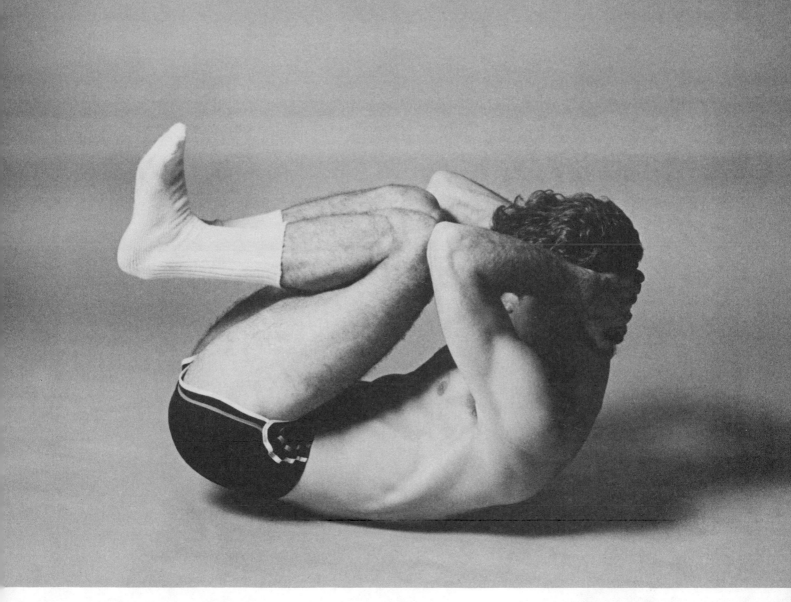

THE CRUNCH

The reason abdominal muscles require so much attention is that normally they aren't worked out very strenuously. Running affects them not nearly enough, for instance, which explains why many joggers are also jigglers. You must concentrate intensely on abdominal muscles to get firm results. Of course, while you're shaping them up, you can also get residual benefits. Here the extras accrue in the upper back area.

Position.

Lie on the floor with your knees bent and your hands behind your neck, fingers interlaced.

Progression.

Keeping your back flat against the floor, slowly draw your knees up as far as you can. Tense your gut and butt while holding this position. Relax them slightly and take a deep breath.

Keeping your knees in that position, slowly raise your back off the ground and try to touch your elbows to your knees. Tighten abdomen and buttocks while holding the position for a second or two.

Lower your back to the floor again but don't rest your head. Keep your knees stationary. Flex, then relax those buttocks and abdominal muscles again.

THE SIDE-UP

What do you think you'll work out next? How about your abdominals? And how about some extra help for your waist? Needless to say, The Side-Up is advantageous for your legs too.

Position.

Lie on your right side, propping your torso on your forearm. Rest your left arm comfortably across your torso so your left palm rests on top of your right hand. Draw your right leg in a bend under your left leg, which should be kept straight with your foot off the ground and flexed.

Progression.

Slowly bending your left knee, bring it as close as possible to your left shoulder by swiveling your leg out and up.

Hold for a moment, tensing your abdominal muscles, then slowly return to the original position. Don't rest your heel on the floor when finished.

Do the same on your other side.

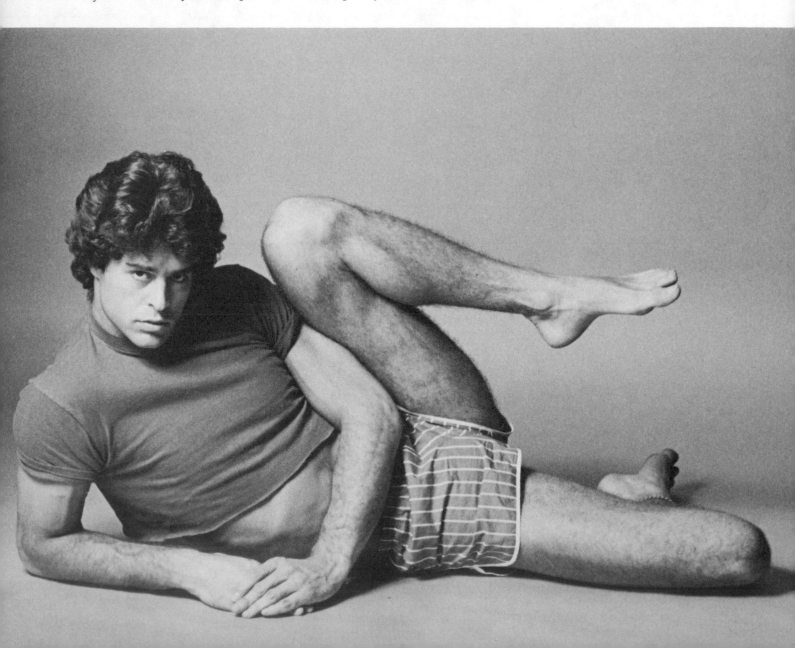

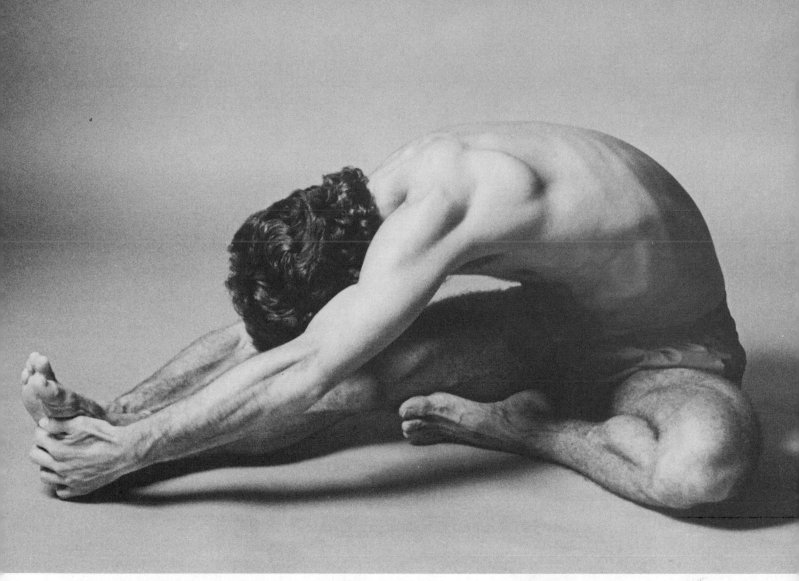

THE "RIDING-THIGH"

This one helps the abdominal muscles too, but that's not its chief intent. As the name suggests, the exercise concentrates on your thighs, particularly the inner parts. But because of the alternating type of movement, it also gets at hamstrings and the buttocks. Overall body tuning occurs as well, adding greatly to total flexibility and coordination. In short, it's damn good.

Position.

Sit on the floor with your back straight, putting the sole of your left foot against your right inner thigh. Your right leg should be straight out in front of you, and your right foot should be flexed, with your toes pointed toward your chest. Rest your hands against your right thigh.

Progression.

Allowing your hands to follow the contours of your leg, slowly bend forward from the waist after taking a deep breath.

Keep bending from the waist with your back straight. At the same time, extend your arms.

Bend and stretch until your forehead rests on your knee (or thereabout) and your fingers touch your toes (if possible). Clasp your toes if you can. Tauten your abdomen and buttocks. Take another deep breath. Hold the position for a moment or two.

Inhale slowly as you gradually resume an upright position.

Do the same on your other side.

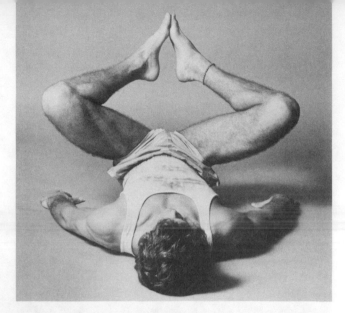

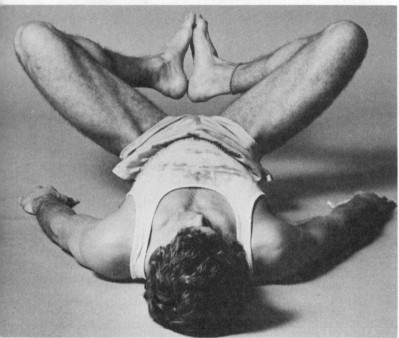

THE "V-FOR-VICTORY"

As your final limbering exercise, this one wraps up the workout by stretching just about all of you. It demands a good measure of practice and patience.

Position.

Lie down with your arms spread a little at your sides and with your back as flat against the floor as possible. With your knees bent, draw your thighs close to your chest.

Progression.

With relaxed shoulders and no arch to the back, flex your feet, then spread your knees until the balls of your feet touch each other.

Reduce the flex to your feet and curve them so your heels also touch.

Breathe deeply. Bend your knees more, lowering your heels, bringing them as close as possible to your crotch. Your legs will form a short and fat diamond.

Gently exhale as you tighten your abdominal and buttocks muscles. Meanwhile, open your legs and spread them into the widest V you can in a lateral fashion, as if opening a book.

Take another deep breath and return your legs straight up at a perpendicular angle to your torso.

Release your breath and tense your butt and gut for a moment.

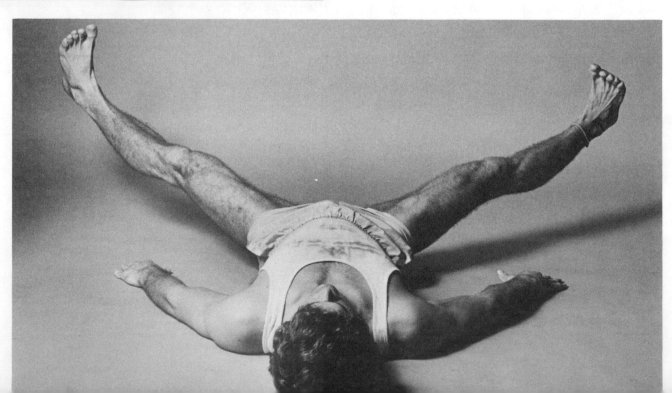

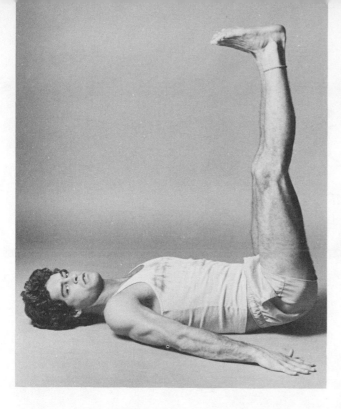

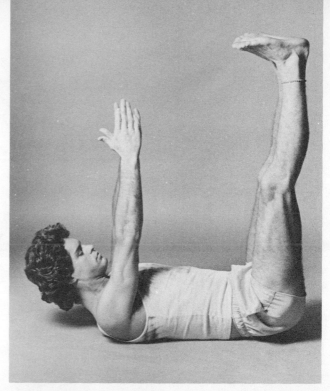

Keeping your legs straight up, raise your arms and stretch them parallel to your legs toward the ceiling.

Bend your knees and lower your thighs toward your chest, clasping your shins when they come within reach. Pull your shins until your thighs and chest compress tightly, as in The Chest/Thigh Embrace (page 67).

Return your feet to the floor, bending your knees. Place your hands crossed on your belly.

Lift your pelvis off the floor. Breathe deeply.

Exhale as you lower your pelvis to the floor.

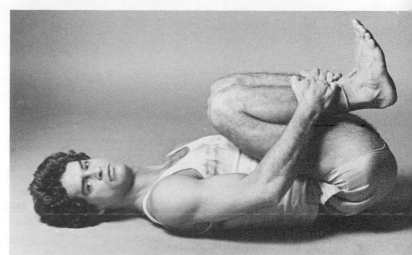

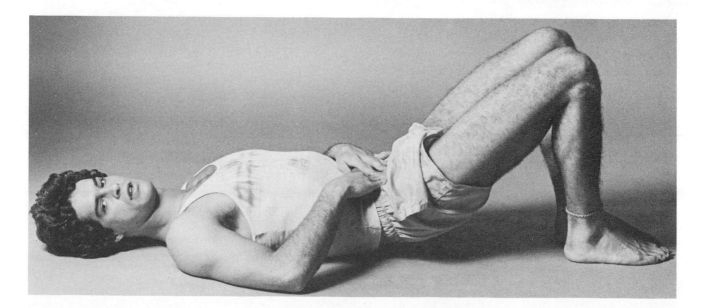

CHAPTER 6

STEPPING LIVELY

ON AND ON

If you've clocked yourself well during your daily limbering routine, by the time you're ready to shift into the maintenance phase of your workout—which will alternate days with your building exercises—you should feel a healthy rush through your body. You should be perspiring, but not profusely. Your face should be pink with vigor, not flushed from exhaustion.

Naturally, as you move onward in your shaping-up program, your performance will improve, and so will your capacity for more strenuous workouts with less of a drain on your system. Then your body will bristle with well-being. And you'll also be that much closer to realizing your ultimate goal of shaping up.

Although it will take some time and patience before you reach that plateau, you should feel close to your physical peak immediately before aerobic concentration, well lubricated and ready to surge.

While aerobics are the backbone of your working-out plan, conceptually they are amazingly simple. Whereas you must go through a whole series of different movements to promote flexibility or to enhance your musculature, you truthfully need do only one among various maintenance exercises—such as running or cycling, swimming or rowing—to raise your aerobic capabilities. And your choice of activities is extremely wide when your aim is aerobic fitness. As long as you gradually—and safely—push your heart to do more and more, it virtually doesn't matter how you do it. Freedom of choice is alive and well in aerobics.

It's not mandatory that you do all the specified maintenance exercises. Any one of them performed regularly and heartily will goose up your cardiovascular system. But just for the hell of it, why not give each a trial run? You'll never know if you truly prefer Bumping to Fancy Stepping unless you experiment. And experimentation is the spice of working out.

Your eventual goal is to go nonstop from limbering into maintenance exercises every other day for a total of twenty to thirty minutes each session, sustaining your heartbeat safely below your maximum. *Don't ever push beyond that.* For now, though, don't even aspire that high; gradually increase your aerobic demands by a minute or two each week, starting out with no more than a ten-minute cardiovascular

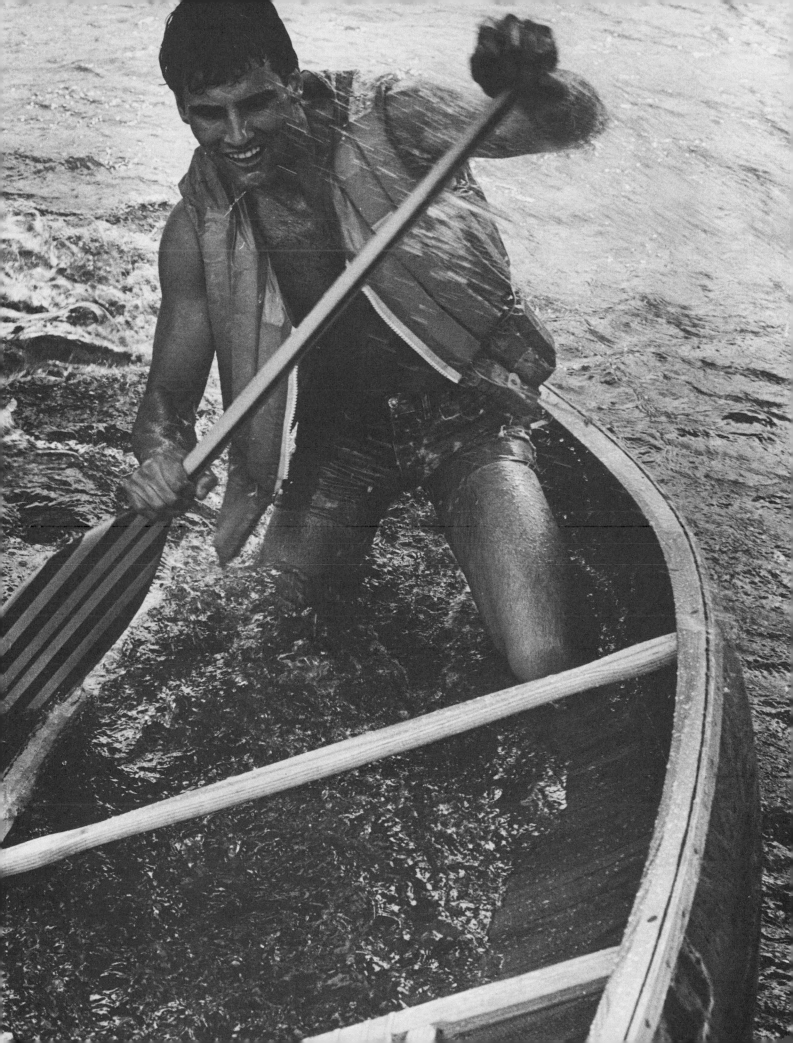

workout unless you're already in excellent shape or unless circumstances are exceptional (see Chapter 8).

During your maintenance sessions, stay motivated by *picturing* and *feeling* what's happening with your body. Keep thinking about where you're heading.

The great advantage of the exercises cited is that they can be performed indoors regardless of the weather—as opposed to cycling or running—and with minimal special facilities—unlike swimming. And they're greatly more effective than team sports. To get the most out of a workout, you supply the labor.

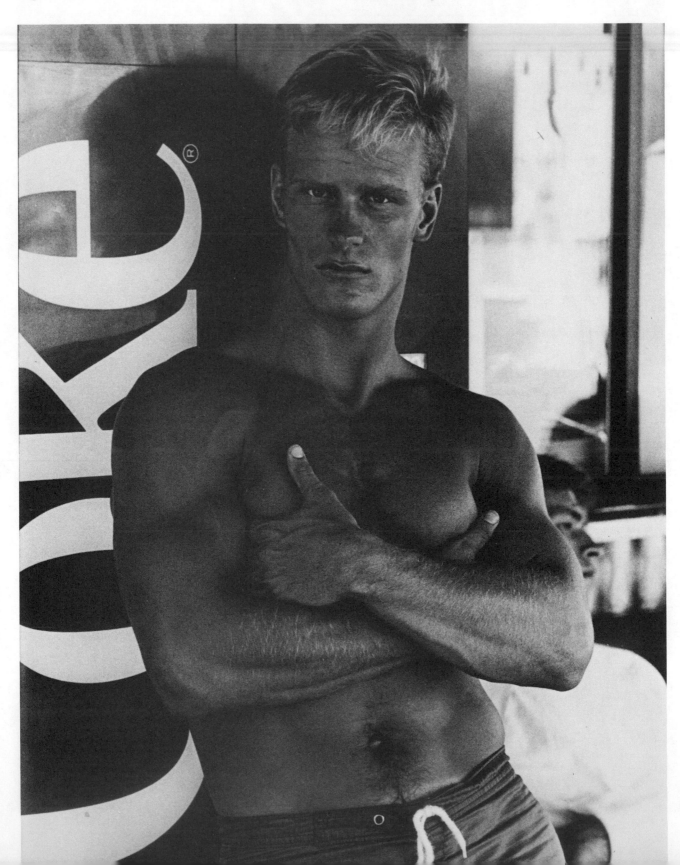

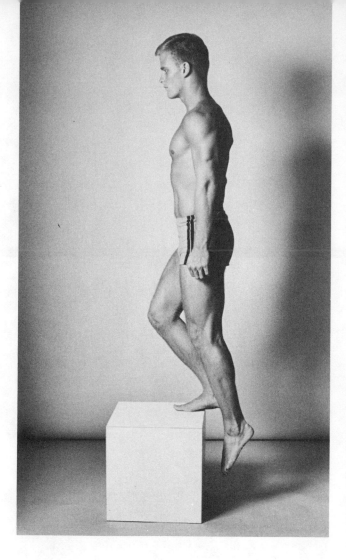
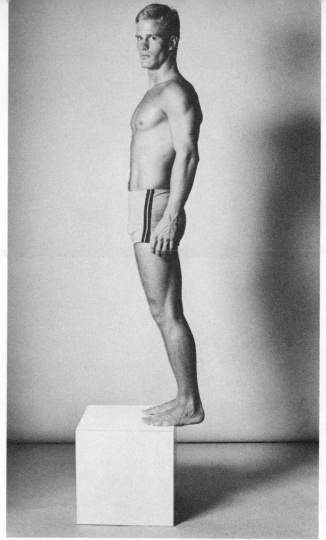

BOXING

Considering some of the high jinks you put yourself through while stretching, this aerobic may seem like pretty tame stuff. A killer it's not, but it does what's necessary by raising your heartbeat and keeping it raised throughout the duration of the exercise. Boxing is also a good way to tone your thighs, firm your buttocks.

If you have an 18-inch cube, you won't need to improvise with stairs or stepladders, which force you to contort your body to get the work done. Keeping your movements rhythmic and regular is essential.

Boxing's value as an aerobic underscores the importance of walking. A good way to prepare yourself for cardiovascular effort is to walk and walk some more for a week or two before even initiating any systematic aerobic workout. If you keep walk-

ing a lot after going full-steam into your workout, so much the better.

Position.

Stand before an 18-inch cube with your back straight, your feet fairly close together and your arms hanging loosely at your sides.

Progression.

Without bending or raising your arms, lift your right foot and put the ball of that foot—*not* your entire foot—over the edge of the cube.

Step up, bringing your left foot beside your right one.

Step down with your right foot, leaving your left one on the edge of the cube.

Now bring your left foot down to the original position.

Repeat, starting this time with your left foot.

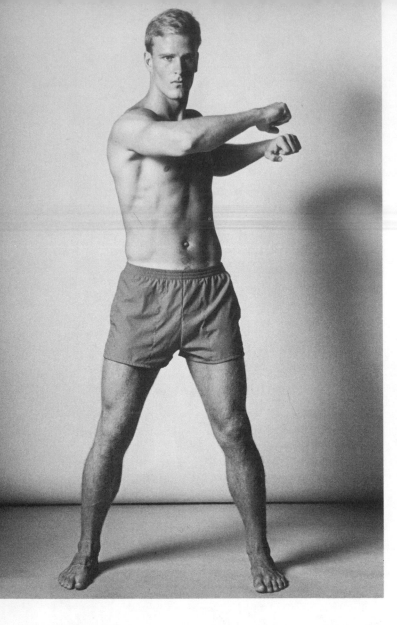
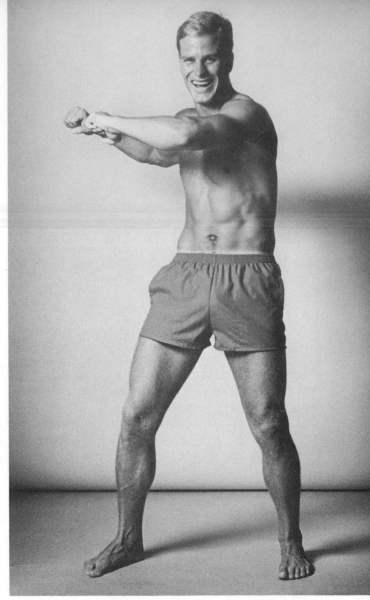

TWISTING

This one is so much fun you might think it's a game, not an exercise. Remember: Exercise is not torture. While you're getting your jollies—and raising your heartbeat—you're also working out your torso against the resistance of your lower body. The whole idea is to twist quickly. If you're too lackadaisical, you won't tax your cardiovascular system, and that's your primary goal. Of course, when first beginning, don't attempt to be a dervish.

Position.

With your feet wide apart and flat on the floor, bend your knees slightly to "lock in" your hips.

(You want to keep your hips stationary throughout this one.) Raise your arms and bend your elbows so they are level with your chest. Your forearms should be parallel to the floor.

Progression.

While keeping your face forward and your hips immovable, swing your right shoulder forward and around toward the left as far as possible while swinging your left shoulder back. Don't move your hips.

Twist back, now swinging your left shoulder as far as possible to the right.

Twist back and forth rapidly but rhythmically.

If you like—or have exhibitionistic tendencies—add a wicked "bump-and-grind" as a final fillip.

SWINGING

Time to serious up a little. Although this exercise appears to be a standard calisthenic, by remaining bent over you will place extra demands on your cardiovascular system as you repeat the specified movements. Simultaneously, your neck, shoulders, waist, lower back, calves, and hamstrings are all getting a lesson in endurance. Once again, your pace must be fairly brisk.

Position.

Stand with your legs widely spread, feet flat on the floor.

Progression.

Bending at the waist and rotating your torso so your shoulders are in parallel alignment with your left leg, extend your right hand—keeping your arm straight—until your fingertips touch your left toes. Don't bend your knees unless absolutely necessary. Simultaneously swing your left arm up so it is perpendicular to the floor and your fingers are pointing straight at the ceiling. As you swing your arms, turn your head so you are gazing over your shoulder behind you at an upward angle.

Staying bent at the waist, reverse the swing of your arms, rotating your torso, so that your left fingers touch your right toes. As you raise your right arm, don't forget to angle your head with an upward glance in the same direction.

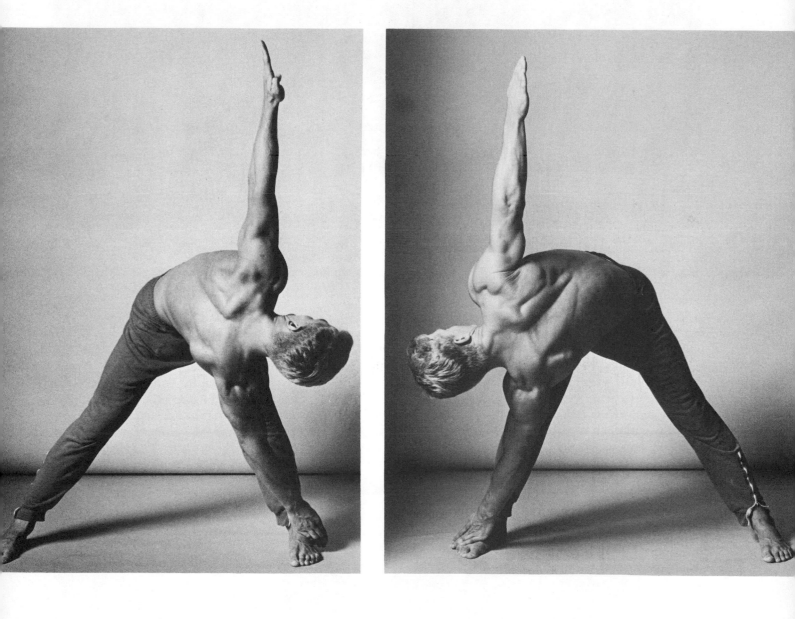

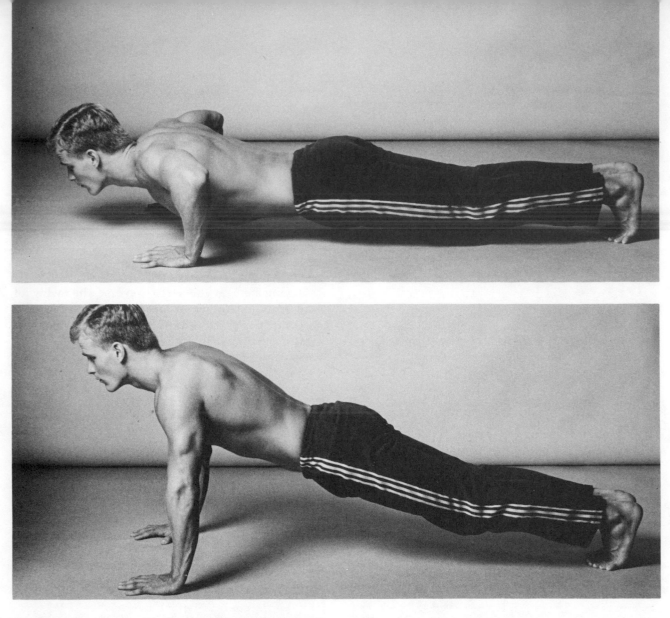

PUSHING

Here is another exercise that bridges calisthenics and aerobics. A brisk pace and constant repetition without any rest time are imperative for cardiovascular benefit.

In all likelihood, you won't choose to spend a full twenty minutes doing push-ups to qualify for your maintenance activity. Not only would that be boring, it could also feel debilitating. But a couple of minutes of push-ups sandwiched between other aerobic movements will also tone up your chest, your shoulders, and particularly your triceps. It pays to concentrate on your breathing patterns while Pushing.

Position.

Lie face down, bending your elbows so your arms can rest, palms on the floor, on either side of your chest. Your fingers should be pointed forward. Your toes should be bent so they are on the floor and your heels are raised.

Progression.

Take a deep breath.

As you gently exhale, raise your torso and waist off the ground by pushing against the floor with your hands and arms until your arms are straight. Your back should likewise be straight, not arched.

Inhale as you bend your elbows to lower your body, maintaining a straight back. Stop a few inches before your torso touches the floor.

Exhale as you push off again.

TRACKING

Because of the compressed lunges involved, this is a highly concentrated aerobic, *not* to be performed for extended periods without interruption. When you use it as part of a maintenance routine, intersperse it between other movements—such as Boxing or Twisting—that will allow your heartbeat to slow a little, though without returning to at-rest normality. But don't prolong this slight breather or considerable aerobic benefit will be lost.

Position.

On your hands and knees, bring your right foot forward so your thigh rests against the right side of your chest and your toes are almost directly below your bent right knee. Extend your left leg out behind you with barely a bend at the knee so that your weight is balanced between the toes of your right and left feet. Use the palms of your hands (positioned in front of your right foot) and your straight arms for additional support. Now try to flatten your right foot against the floor, stretching your Achilles tendon. (You may not be able to complete this difficult movement initially.)

Progression.

Inhale deeply.

With a little bounce to build momentum, quickly reverse the positioning of your right and left feet, landing on your toes.

Always bring the forward foot as far forward as possible while extending the back foot as far backward as you can.

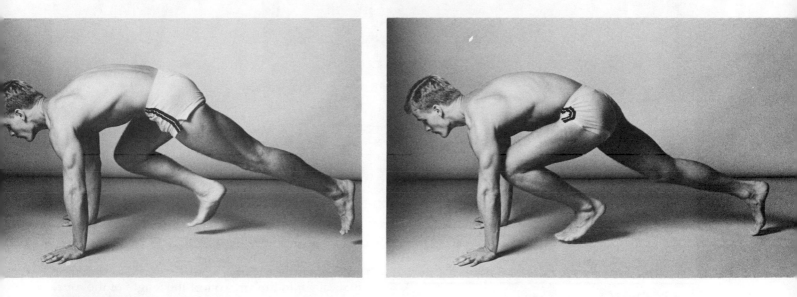

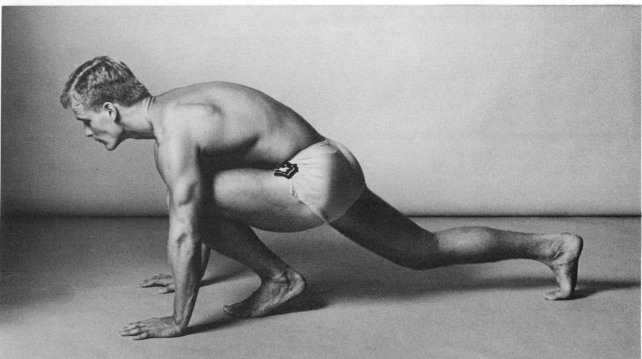

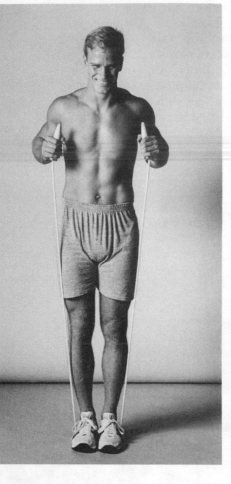
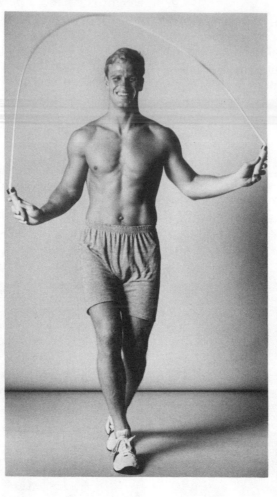
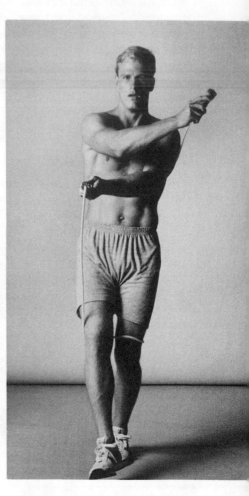

SKIPPING

Although skipping rope seems child's play, like Tracking it accelerates your heartbeat very rapidly —too rapidly if you're not in good shape and you skip to beat the band. You should skip for only a minute or two when starting out, gradually increasing your time twirling the rope up to five minutes. Then slow your heart down a bit with a less strenuous exercise for a couple of minutes before taking up the rope again. Even when you're in superb shape, don't go into Skipping in a marathon fashion.

Position.

How you jump the rope—on both feet or only one—is secondary in importance to the cardiovascular boost. But for efficiency's sake, don't leap dramatically into the air. To test the length of the rope, stand on its center and raise the ends toward your armpits. If that's where the ends of the rope rest— near your armpits—swell.

Progression.

Holding the ends of the rope in both hands, make sure the loop of the rope is behind your heels.

With a swift lift and twirl of the wrists, swing the rope over the back of your head so it comes around toward your feet.

Skip a couple of inches off the floor as the rope passes under your feet. Hopefully, when you alight on the balls of your feet, the rope will already have passed under them.

With minimal flapping, keep the rope rotating and keep skipping it.

Disentangle as necessary.

FANCY STEPPING

You don't need to do this one "in place." If the spirit moves you, dash outside and actually cover ground.

As in all the preceding maintenance exercises, this final one isn't really much better at augmenting aerobic fitness than running, cycling, swimming, or any other of the aerobic sports. On the other hand, Fancy Stepping is better at developing coordination, speed, and endurance than most of them simply because it's more intensive. Being intensive, Fancy Stepping is also taxing. But once you've heightened your cardiovascular capabilities, you could do this one for hours on end without detriment. If that's your idea of a wonderful day, so be it. Some might prefer stepping out in more fanciful directions.

Position.

Stand with your back straight and your legs slightly spread, bouncing a bit on the balls of your feet.

Progression.

Start running in place, swinging your bent-at-the-elbow left arm forward, your bent-at-the-elbow right arm backward, as you lift your right leg, bringing your knee as close as possible to your chest.

Continue running in place, reversing arms and legs, always landing on the balls of your feet.

Raise your knees progressively higher and higher while accelerating your pace.

Breathe deeply as you persist in your Fancy Stepping.

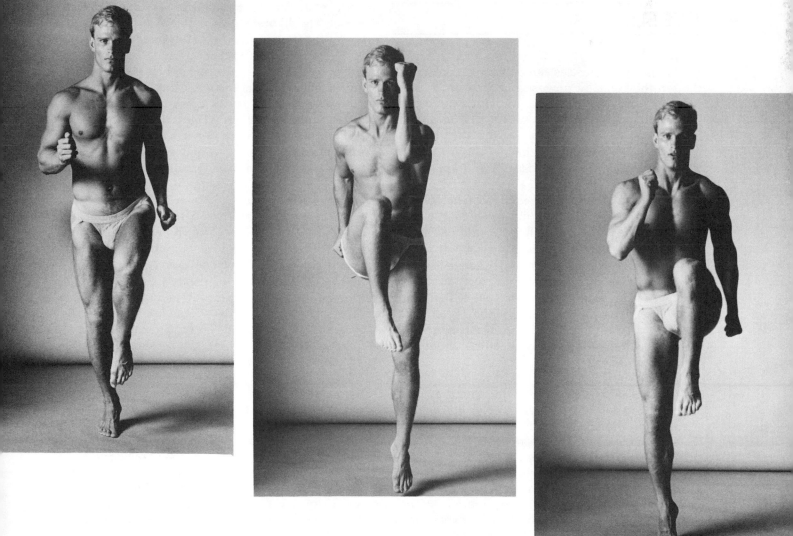

CHAPTER 7

CLOSE INSPECTION

EYEFULS

Well-delineated muscles can be very deceptive. Although they usually suggest a healthy body, that's not necessarily the truth: A guy with a marbleized physique could be a heartbeat away from a heart attack if he isn't aerobically fit. But the strongest cardiovascular system imaginable doesn't guarantee an attractive physique. Health and appearance are not one and the same.

Unless your occupation requires powerful muscles, admit to yourself from the outset that the only reason to add musculature to your frame is to look better. If you face this fact now, you won't waste a lot of psychic energy inventing other reasons for entering the building phase of your workout. Admit it, you're vain. And what's wrong with that? Nothing. (You're also a lot more honest than fellows who insist they're building muscles for reasons of health. There's nothing inherently healthy about pronounced muscles.)

As you know, you should always precede progressive-resistance activities with tuning and limbering exercises. (As you also know, you perform aerobics on the off-days when you're not involved in building exercises.) When you're prepared to enter the building stage, your entire body—and mind—should feel finely tuned. If you're overly tired, rest a bit to collect yourself. There's nothing to be gained by storming on, and there could be a lot to lose. Although you must literally exhaust your muscles to receive any gain from progressive resis-

tance, your muscles must never be exhausted at the outset: They'll break down, not build up. To repeat an oft-repeated sentiment: It's better to be a cunning tortoise than a foolish hare.

Most building exercises incorporate weights. Lifting weights to promote muscle mass involves either increasing the number of times you repeat the exercise with the same weight, or increasing the amount of weight while performing the exercise the same number of times. As time goes by, should you desire even more brimming muscles, you will have to increase both the number of repetitions *and* the amounts of weight.

Building musculature is a more individual process than warming up or stretching, even than aerobics. To maximize your genetic physical potential, you should do at least one exercise per section— that is, at least one Neck exercise, one Shoulder exercise, et cetera—several times during your workout. That way you'll see overall improvement. But if you have specific aims—say you want to give the impression of possessing wider shoulders—then you'll supplement the workout with additional specific exercises (in this instance, the other two Shoulder exercises listed). Three exercises are given for every body part, excepting the Arms, which get five exercises of their own.

Since the principal goal of your workout is to attain a more attractive physique generally, the building exercises touch upon all your body zones, ignoring the head (you wouldn't want to be called a musclehead), starting at the neck, and progressing down to your calves (who desires well-muscled ankles?) for ease of reference. When actually exe-

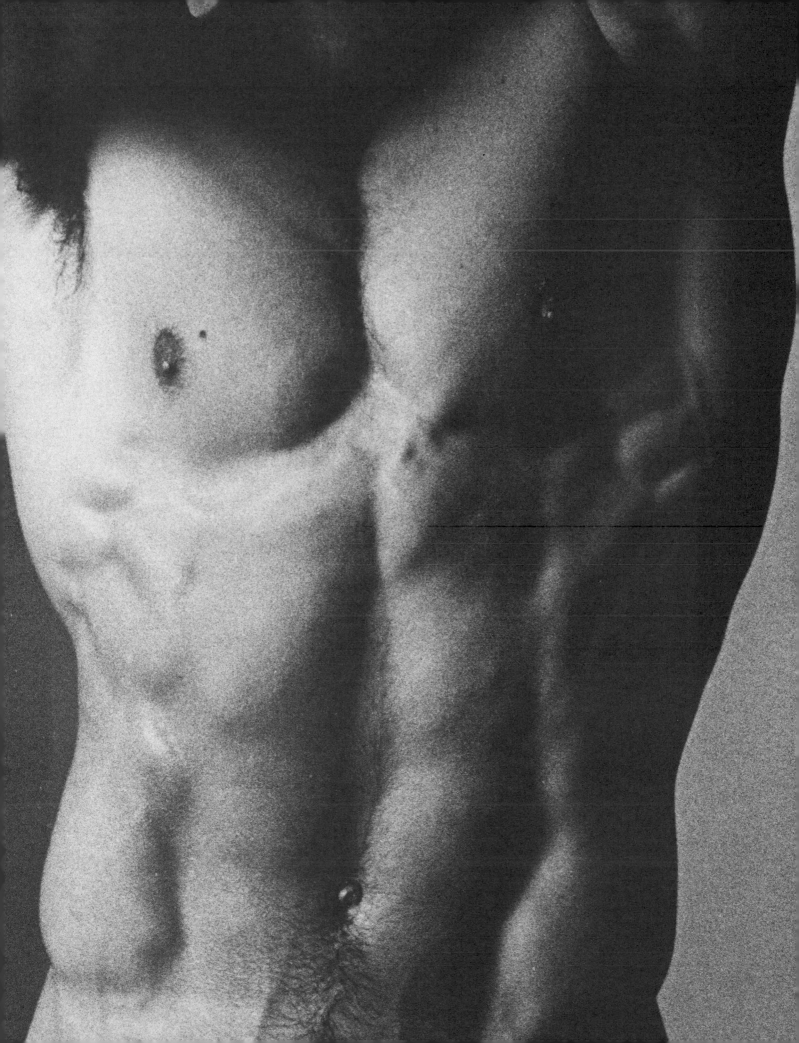

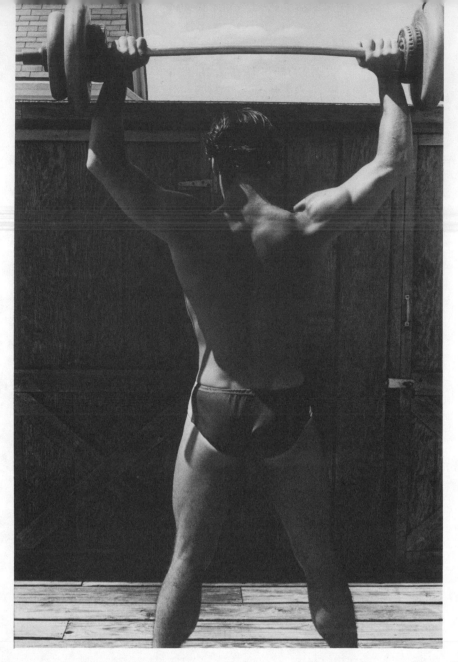

cuting the exercises, you might prefer to do them in a different sequence. To make that decision, check out Chapter 8 for special considerations. For now, simply read through the exercises several times so you will be familiar with their scope.

Just to keep the terminology straight: A rep (or repetition) refers to all the movements involved in the execution of an exercise from start to finish, while a set is the specified number of times an exercise (rep) is executed start to finish, one after another, without any rest time.

When dealing with weights, resist the temptation to take on too much. Remember, you'll be lifting weights repetitiously over a whole series of exercises. You have to save some energy reserve for the finale.

Gauging how heavy or light your weights should be is tricky. If you lift insufficient weight, you're not spurring your muscles to enlarge. If you heave too much, you'll tire too early and you'll risk injury. The only way to determine the correct weight is to experiment. If you can breeze through several reps, you're being too easy on yourself. If you feel as if you'll have to give up entirely after only one attempt, you're asking too much of yourself. For now.

Depending upon your current strength, you may start out with one rep constituting a set. Or, if you're already quite strong, your sets might consist of five reps. *You* make the difference: In working out wisely, there's no such animal as a universal beginning stage; but there is a beginning plateau *for you.*

As you proceed with progressive-resistance exercises, your muscularity will increase and so will your endurance. Later on, you'll be handling heavier weights more readily than you can manipulate lighter ones now. In effect, the more you work out, the easier the process becomes. The fact that the work keeps growing less arduous is your reason for working ever harder.

Generally, weight-training sessions are measured not in minutes but by the number of sets executed. You're seldom working against a clock; you're working against yourself. For now, however, unless you're an excellent specimen, plan to work out with weights for only ten minutes or so every other day for two weeks, gradually extending your sessions. Your eventual goal should be a half to a full hour of progressive resistance, more if you possess the time and inclination, gradually increasing the number of reps per set and/or the number of sets performed. (Under certain circumstances, you should delay building exercises until well under way in limbering and maintenance sessions. See Chapter 8 for details.) If you're sensible and cautious, there's no reason that somewhere down the road you can't do building exercises for two hours on alternate days. On the other hand, there's no reason for you to expend that amount of time unless you want to; a half-hour every other day will make an extraordinary visible difference. More time, more rewards.

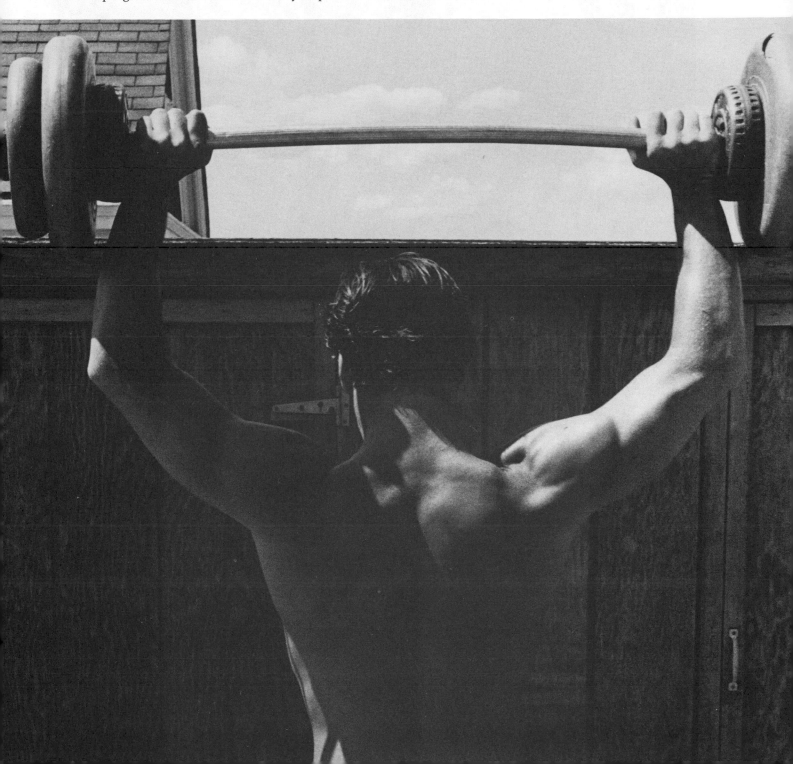

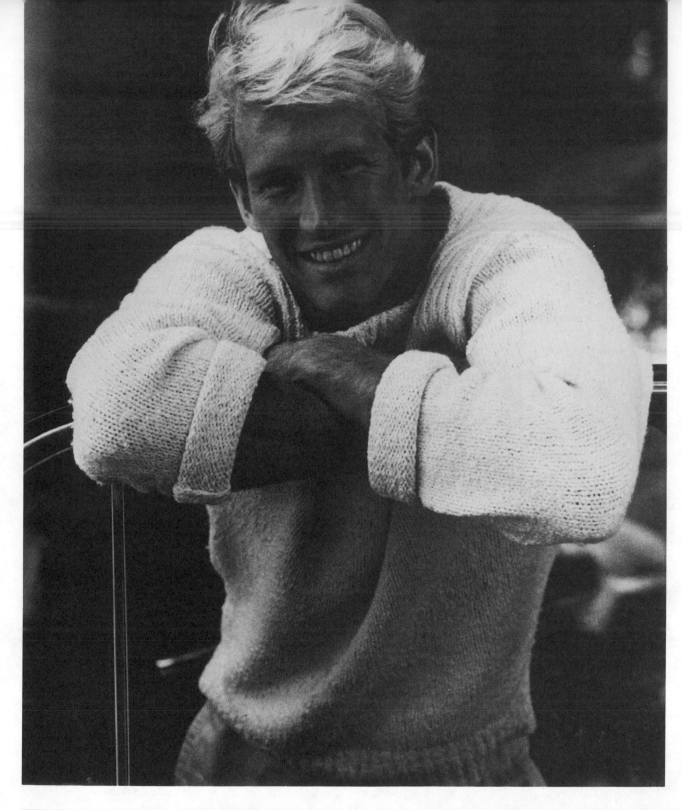

THE NECK

It's not easy to isolate the neck muscles and work out only them. They are intimately bound to the shoulder and upper back muscles, especially the trapezius, which rests on either side of the neck at the top of the back. To attain a more powerful-look-ing neck, concentrate on strengthening the trapezius. Shrugging movements are particularly helpful.

The Weighted Shrug is a variation on The Shrug you do as a warm-up with the addition of light dumbbells. The Lift-and-Shrug involves additional back muscles but still does a job on the neck. The Row-Up, one of the most effective exercises for the trapezius, also develops shoulder muscles.

THE WEIGHTED SHRUG

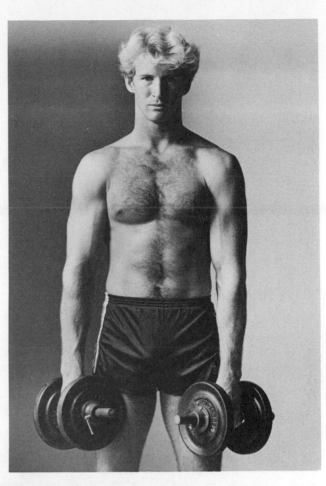

Position.

With a dumbbell in each hand, stand with your arms hanging at your sides, your legs spread to shoulder width.

Progression.

Inhale as you slowly lift your shoulders in an exaggerated shrug, as if you were trying to catch your neck in a vise between your shoulders.

Exhale as you slowly drop your shoulders to the original position.

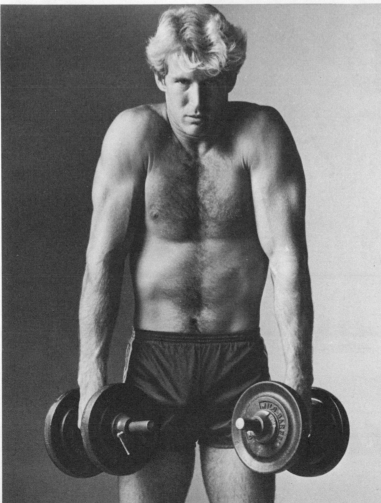

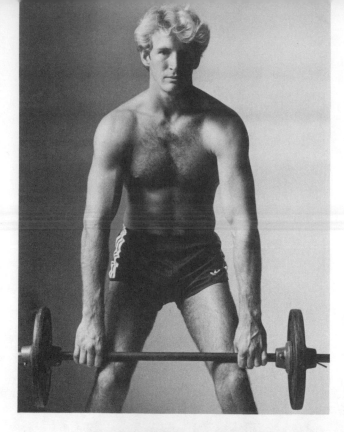

THE LIFT-AND-SHRUG

Position.

With a barbell between your hands in an overhand grip (with your palms pointed in toward your body) and with your knees slightly bent, rest the barbell three or four inches above your kneecaps, bending forward a little at the waist.

Progression.

Inhale.

Exhale as you slowly and smoothly stand up straight until your back is erect and your chin level.

Inhale as you slowly shrug, giving your shoulders an extra-good lift.

Exhale as you slowly lower your shoulders.

Return the barbell to the above-the-kneecap position.

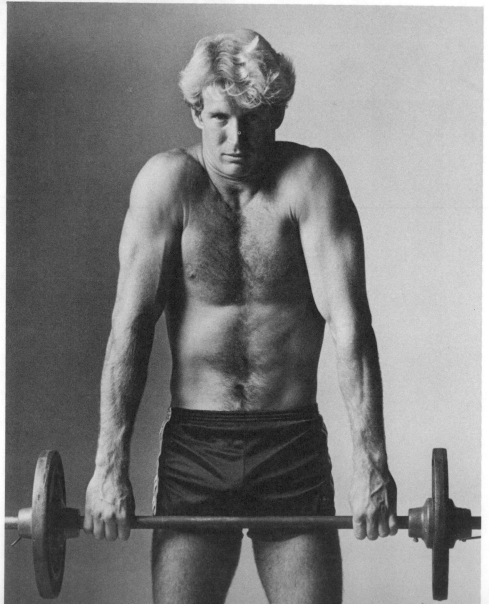

THE ROW-UP

Position.

With an overhand grip, clasp a barbell and hold it about a foot away from the front of your thighs. Your feet should be spread to shoulder width.

Progression.

Inhaling, draw the barbell up to your chin. Exhaling, slowly return it to the original position.

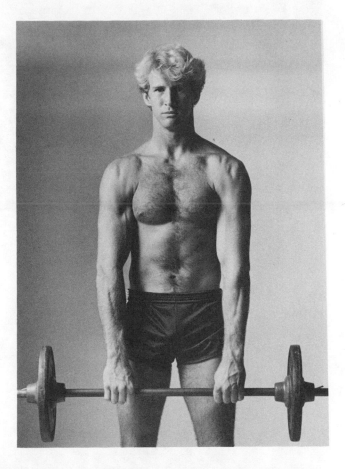

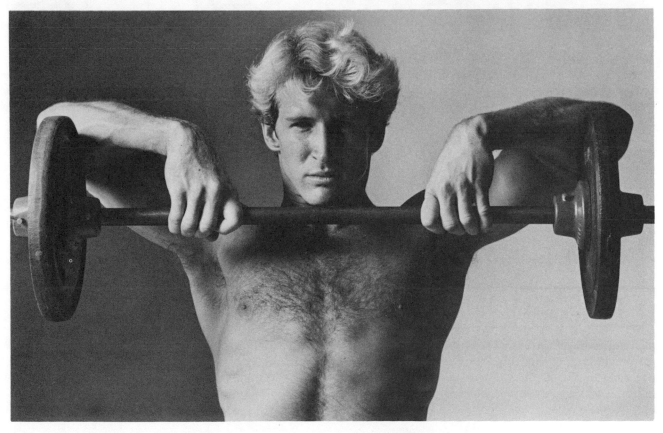

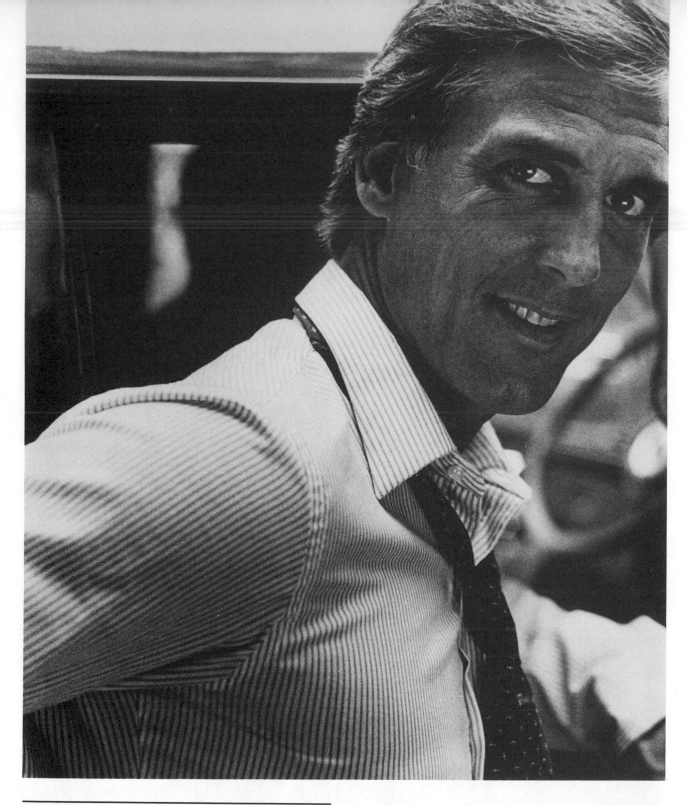

THE SHOULDERS

As you worked on your neck, you simultaneously zeroed in on the trapezius. Your deltoids—the muscle caps in the front and rear over your shoulder joints—are the remaining shoulder muscles requiring attention.

The Dip doesn't involve weights other than the resistance of your body. Even so, it's extremely effective in directly working out your shoulders, not to mention your triceps (which back up your biceps). The Press-Back uses a barbell to "square off" your deltoids. The Dumb Lat is a dumbbell exercise to contour the shoulders.

THE DIP

Position.

First, position three 18-inch cubes. Two of them should be side by side, about eighteen inches apart, so you could—but won't—set yourself snugly between them. The third cube should be centered between the two about three feet away.

Now, position yourself. With your elbows bent and your arms pushed back, place both your palms on the tops of the side-by-side cubes. Clasp your fingers over the edges for support and leverage. Swing your feet up over the edge of the third cube you're facing.

Progression.

Slowly straightening your arms, lift yourself up in the air until your legs are parallel to the ground.

Inhale as you slowly bend your elbows, lowering yourself until your buttocks nearly touch the ground, exhaling gradually as you dip.

Inhale, then lift yourself once more. Dip again, but don't touch down.

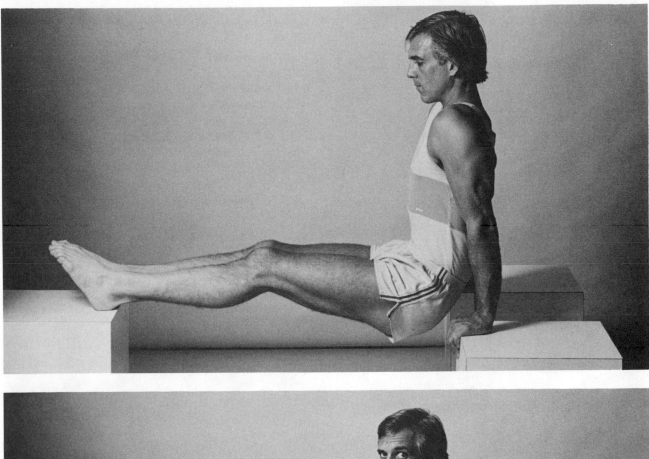

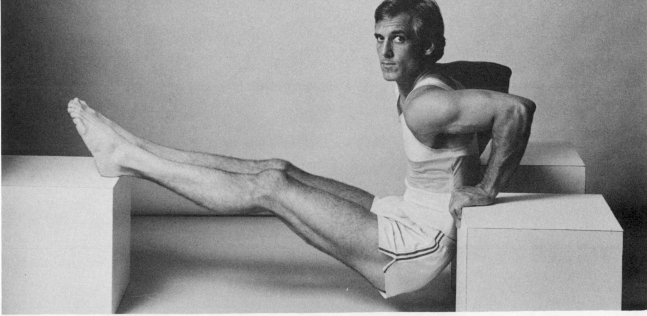

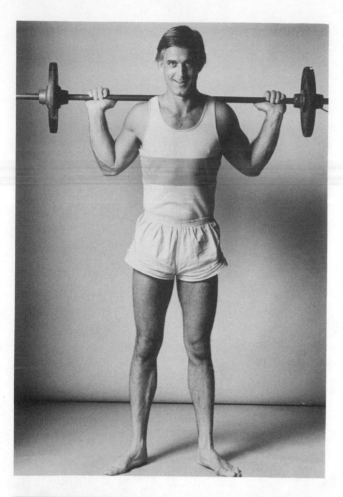

THE PRESS-BACK

Position.

With a barbell resting on your shoulders behind your neck, stand erect with your feet spread shoulder width.

Progression.

Inhaling, lift the barbell straight up—without knocking your noggin—until your arms are almost but not totally straight. (There should be a little bend at the elbows.)

Lower the barbell slowly to the original position, then exhale.

Lift again.

This time when you lower the barbell, don't return it all the way to the shoulders but cut the descent short behind the neck to work on the frontal and lateral deltoids.

Lift again.

Lower the barbell to the shoulders to concentrate on the trapezius and the rear deltoids.

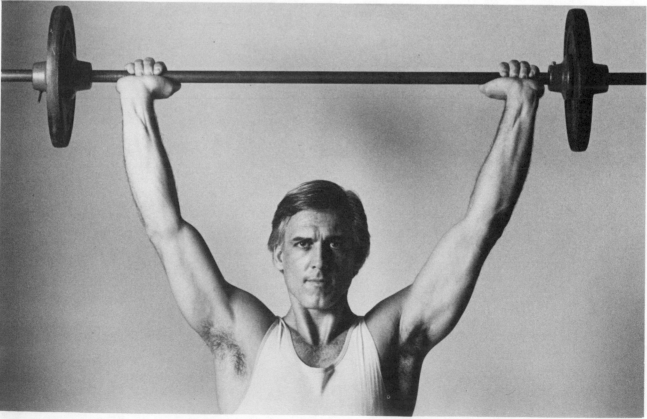

THE DUMB LAT

Position.

Holding dumbbells in the overhand grip, stand straight with your arms hanging and your feet spread slightly.

Progression.

Slowly raise your arms, keeping them straight, until the dumbbells are nearly level with the top of your head. (Be certain you keep your palms pointed downward throughout the lift.)

Slowly lower your arms back to your sides.

To receive optimum benefit for your deltoids, never swoop or swing. The muscle tension that accompanies controlled execution produces the toning.

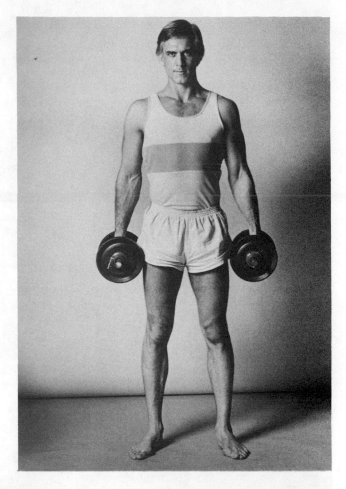

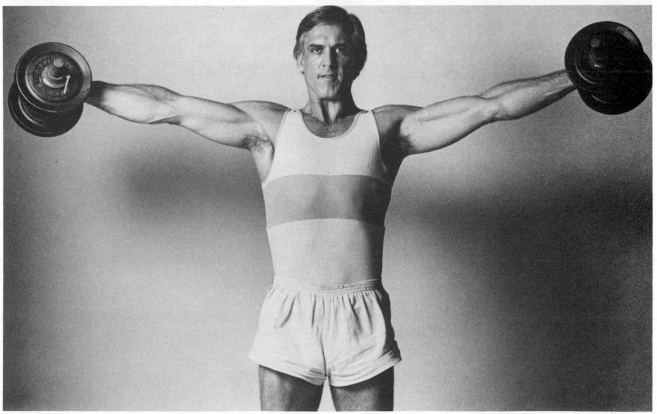

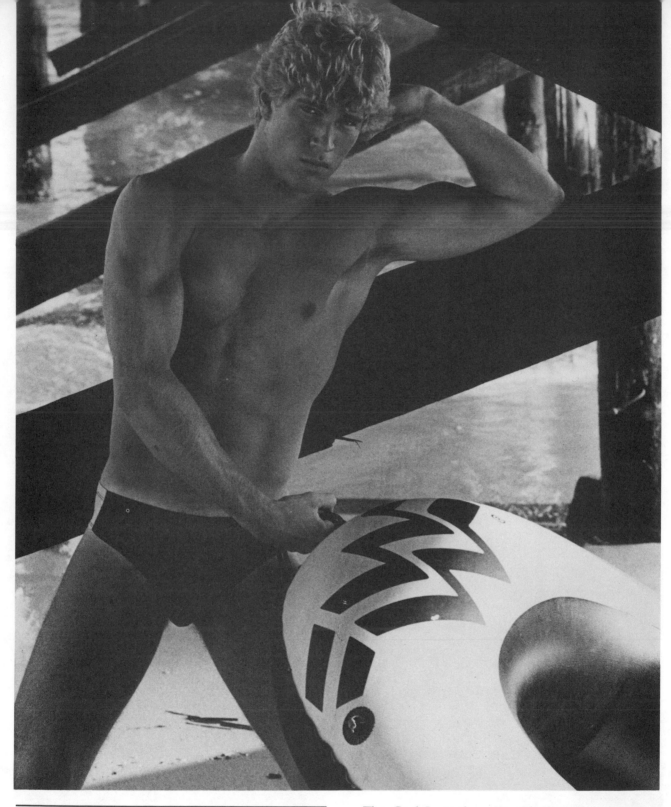

THE ARMS

The strategy for building up arm muscles is straight-forward: Work out the biceps, triceps, and fore-arms, and you're basically set. The "curl" is the major weapon, while "extending" is a good backup.

The Curl I employs dumbbells to build biceps. The Curl II uses a barbell to the same end. The Curl III is yet another biceps builder that also works out the top of the forearms.

The Extension I homes in on the triceps, as does The Extension II.

THE CURL I

Position.

Holding a dumbbell in each hand, stand with your arms hanging at your sides and with your feet slightly spread.

Progression.

Take a deep breath. Raising your elbow a little as you proceed, curl the right dumbbell up (leaving the left arm straight down), turning your wrist so that the end away from your thumb rotates toward your body as you lift the dumbbell in an arc.

Releasing your breath, lower the dumbbell, turning the end closer to your thumb toward your body as you return to the original position.

Repeat with your left arm, turning your wrist so that the end away from your thumb rotates toward your body as you lift the dumbbell in an arc.

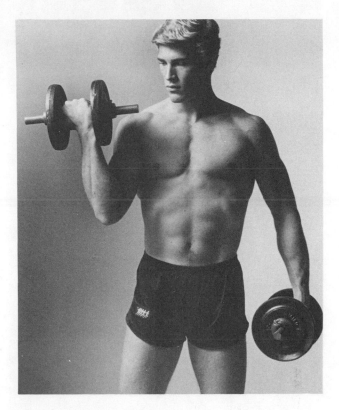

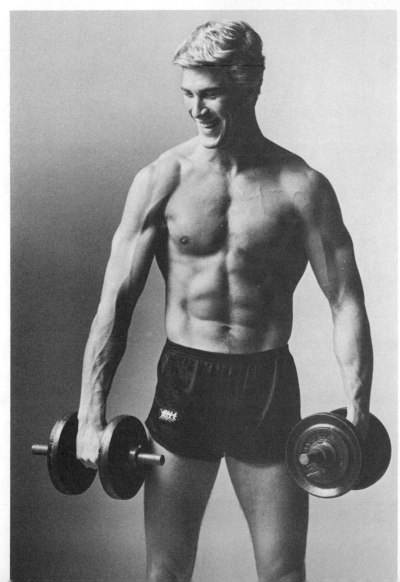

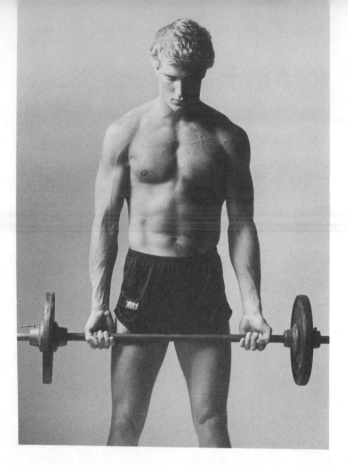

THE CURL II

Position.

Holding the barbell in an underhand grip (palms facing away from the body) with your hands spread to approximately shoulder width, stand upright with your feet slightly spread.

Progression.

As you inhale, keeping your elbows next to your torso, slowly curl the barbell up, moving it in an arc until it is close to your body below your chin.

Slowly reverse the arc, lowering the barbell to the original position, exhaling.

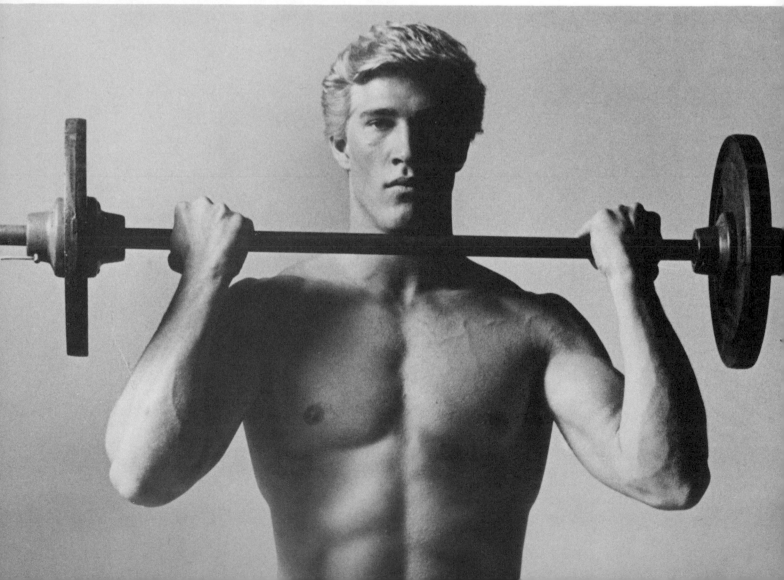

THE CURL III

Position.

Holding the barbell in the overhand grip, stand with your arms straight at your sides and your feet slightly spread.

Progression.

Holding the bar extra firmly to work out the forearms, inhale and slowly curl the barbell upward in an arc by keeping your elbows fairly close to your sides, lifting them only a little as the bar comes parallel to your shoulders so the bar can graze your chin.

Keeping a tight squeeze on the bar, exhale and slowly lower the barbell to the original position.

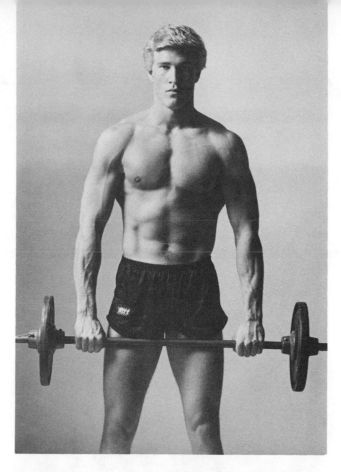

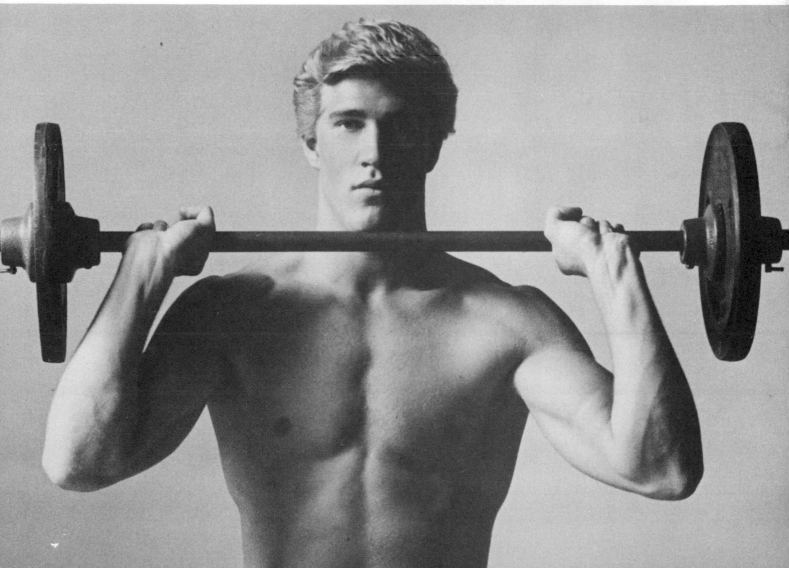

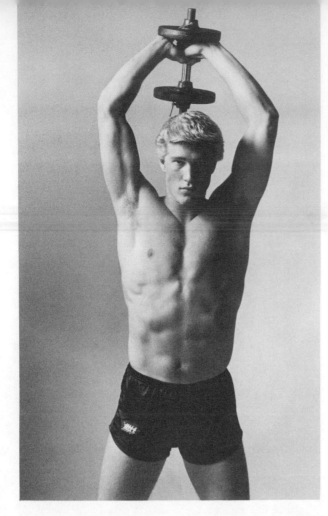

THE EXTENSION I

Position.

Pay close attention to your elbows in this one. Standing straight with your feet spread to shoulder width, clasp a dumbbell at one end with both hands and raise it behind your head so your elbows are at a 45-degree angle to your body in order to work out the triceps completely.

Progression.

Take a breath and slowly lower the dumbbell as far as you can behind you, leaning back slightly.

Slowly return the dumbbell to the original position, releasing your breath.

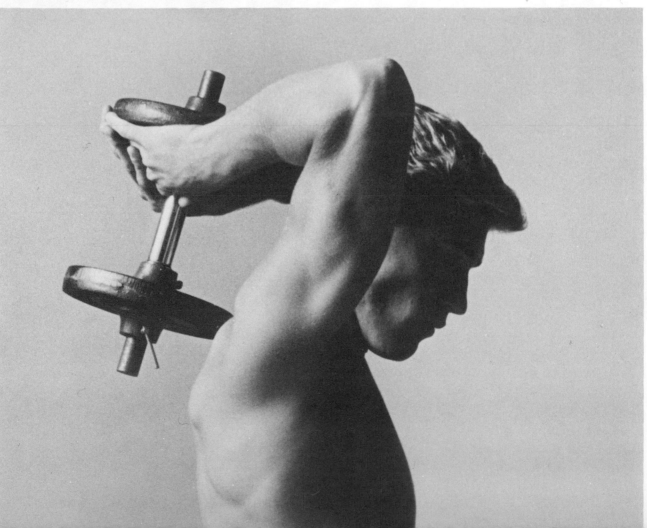

THE EXTENSION II

Position.

Standing with a dumbbell in your right hand, raise it above your head, rotating your elbow close to the back of your head.

Progression.

Keeping your elbow as tight to your head as possible, draw a deep breath, then slowly lower the dumbbell down toward the top of your shoulders and (if possible) beyond to the middle of your back.

Exhaling, slowly straighten your arm, with your elbow still hugging your head, until the dumbbell is overhead again.

Repeat with dumbbell in your left hand.

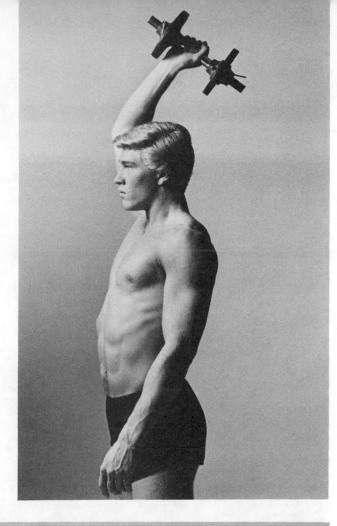

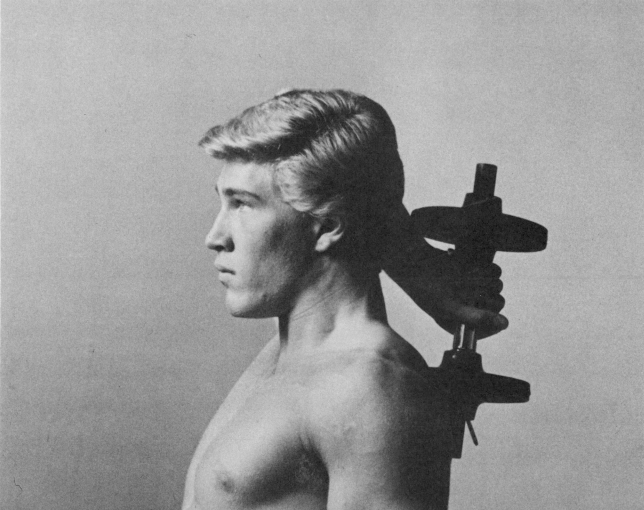

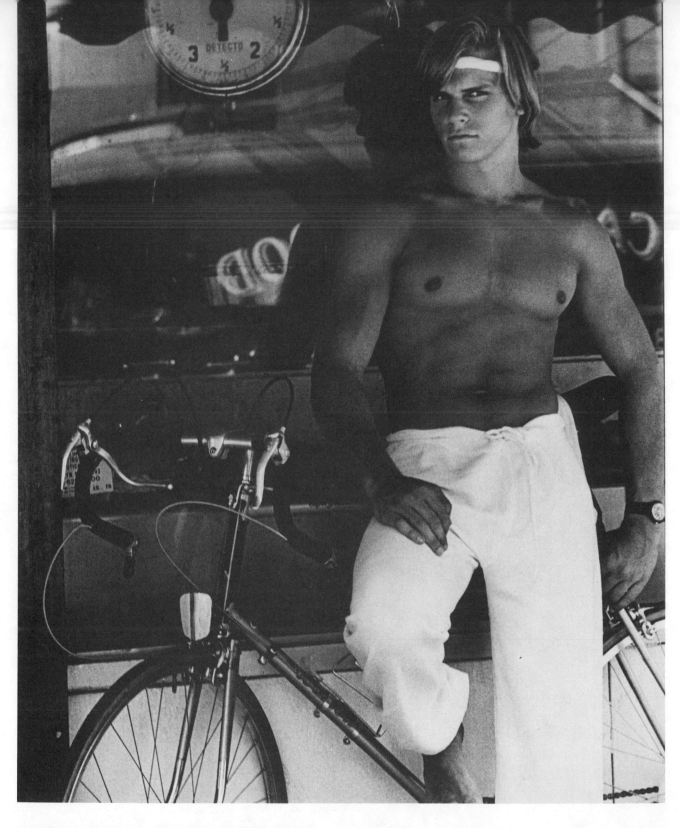

THE CHEST

The most important muscles to develop on the chest for a flattering physique are the pectorals (located between the collarbone and the sternum, also called the breastbone) and the serratus (the group travers-ing the upper torso from the pectorals in front below the armpit to the major muscles of the back).

The Push-Off is a rigorous form of push-up, de-signed to work out the entire chest, also the deltoids and triceps. The Dumb Fly does a great job on the outer pectorals, and The Dumb Over is especially efficacious for the serratus as well as the muscles surrounding the rib cage.

THE PUSH-OFF

Position.

With an 18-inch cube behind you, balancing yourself face down with your hands spread shoulder width on the floor, palms down and fingers forward, swing your feet up on the cube and stretch until your back and your arms are straight.

Progression.

Inhaling deeply, bend your elbows to lower your body so the tip of your chin touches the floor.

Straighten your arms to lift your body until it's parallel to the floor, exhaling when you stop.

Inhale, repeat.

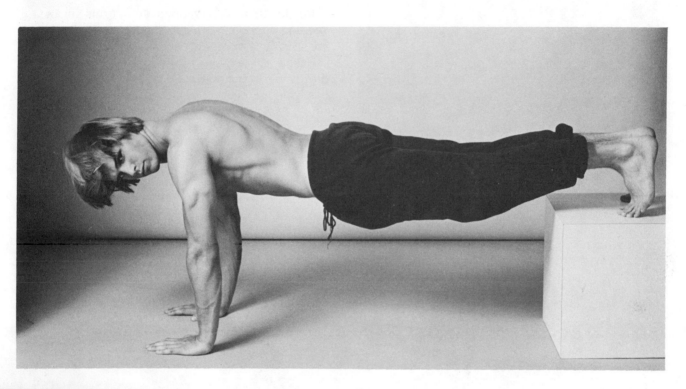

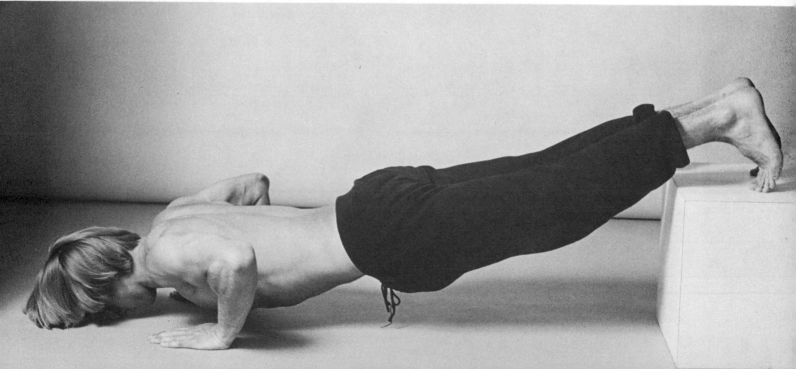

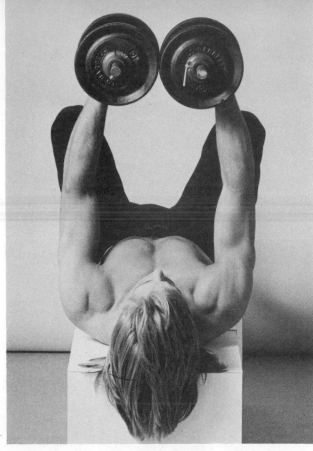

THE DUMB FLY

Position.

Reclining on a bench (or any elevated flat surface), your knees bent and the balls of your feet extending over the end, raise your hands—each holding a dumbbell—over your chest until the dumbbells nearly touch and your arms are almost straight but slightly bent at the elbows.

Progression.

Inhale, then slowly open your arms in an arc, keeping your elbows slightly bent, until your hands are slightly lower than your back.

Exhale as you slowly lift your arms, returning the dumbbells to the original position.

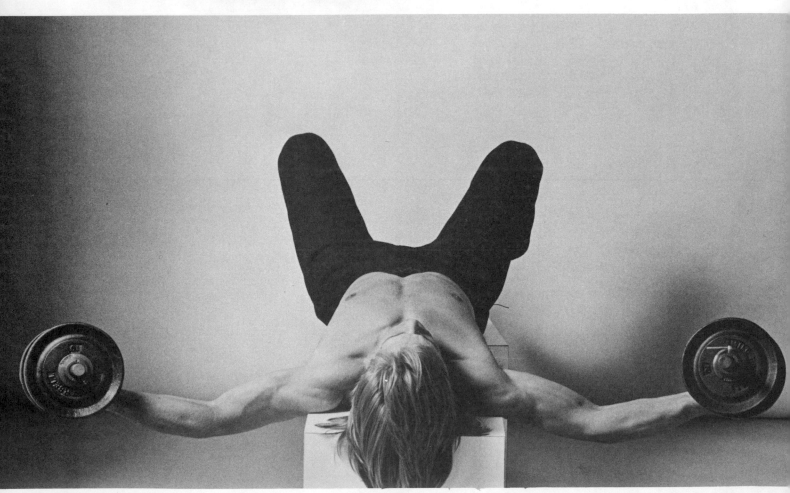

THE DUMB OVER

Position.

With your shoulders resting across a bench, hang your head over one side, extending your legs (ankles together) straight out over the other, your feet flat on the floor if possible. Lift a dumbbell in one hand until you can clasp the end with both hands, then raise it above you until your arms are nearly but not quite straight.

Progression.

Breathing deeply, slowly lower the dumbbell behind your head, extending your arms in an arch, until it almost touches the floor.

Arch your back, puffing your chest.

As you exhale, slowly bring the dumbbell overhead again. Inhale and repeat.

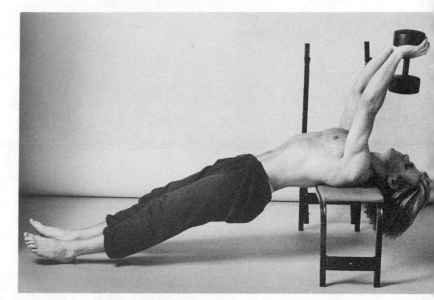

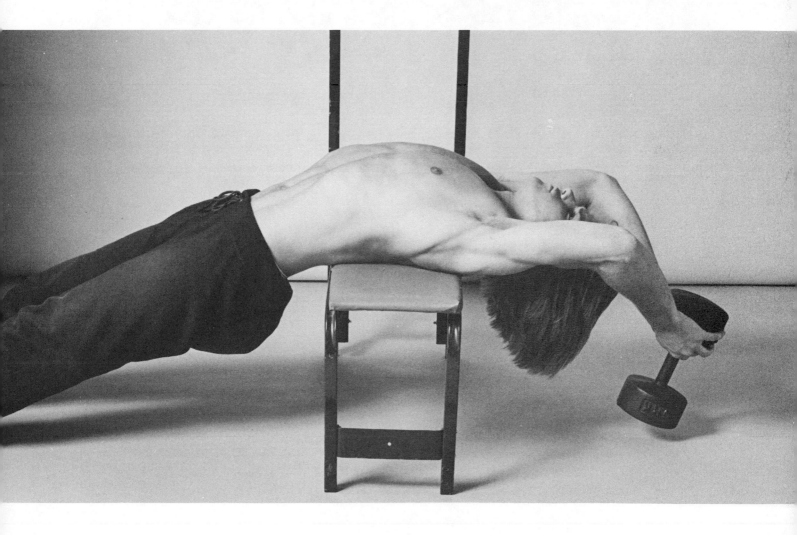

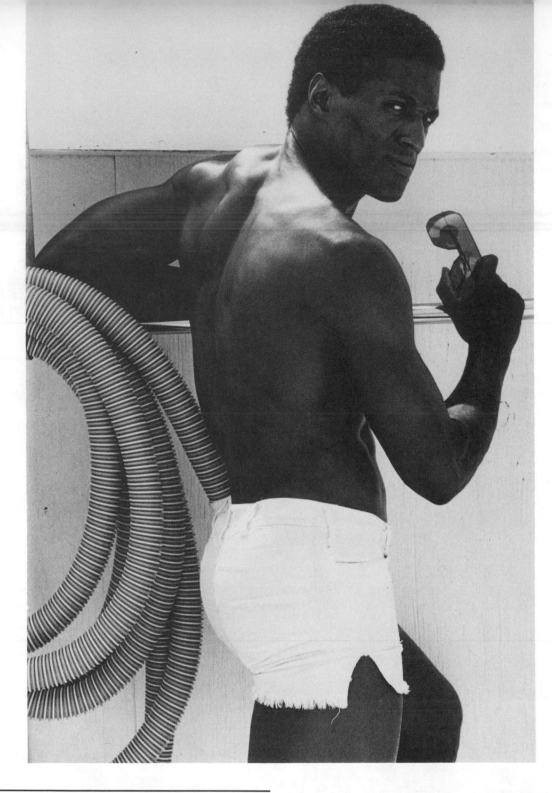

THE BACK

A well-delineated back is impossible if your neck and shoulder muscles aren't effectively built up. Conversely, working on your neck and shoulders gives you a head start on your back muscles.

The back muscles you're particularly interested in are the latissimus dorsi (which extend all the way across the back from the lower spine to your rear shoulders) and the spinal erectors (which go along the lower spine section.)

The Dumb Row is an all-around winner, specifically building up the outer area of the lats while also zeroing in on the lower back. The Row-Down is also excellent for shaping up the back, with particular emphasis on the lower back without cheating the upper part. The Deadlift goes beyond the back (giving the upper portion an extra-good workout) and contributes to overall strength and endurance.

THE DUMB ROW

Position.

Standing before a bench with your feet widely spread (about two feet apart), with your knees bending a little, lean forward and place your left hand on the bench. Use your left arm for support, and bend your elbow to keep your chest parallel to the floor. Clasp a dumbbell in your right hand.

Progression.

Inhale as you raise the dumbbell until it touches your chest.

Exhaling, lower the dumbbell to the floor without changing the position of your back.

Do the same with your other arm.

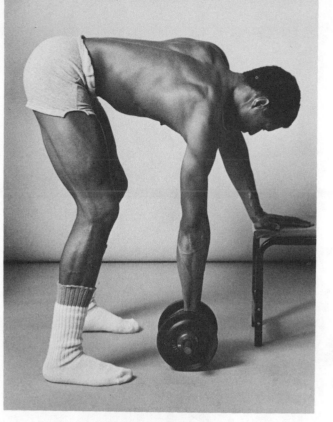

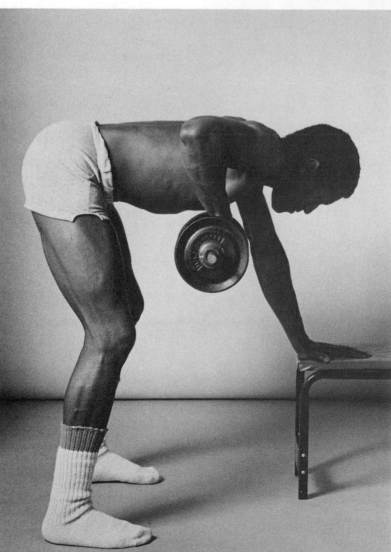

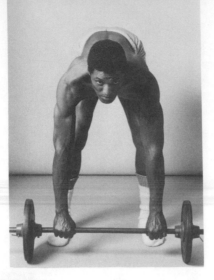

THE ROW-DOWN

Position.

Standing on the floor with your feet spread shoulder width, bend over (keeping your knees bent a little) until your chest is parallel to the floor. Clasp the barbell in the overhand grip with your hands spread a bit wider than shoulder width.

Progression.

Inhale, then draw the barbell up until it touches your chest. Do not raise your back.

Exhale, then slowly lower the barbell.

This time, as you raise the barbell after inhaling, raise your upper body as you lift the barbell, pulling it to touch the bottom of your rib cage. By this change of position, instead of concentrating primarily on the lats as you did when remaining bent at the waist, you are putting more emphasis on the spinal erectors *and* trapezius.

Exhale, lowering the barbell and your torso as well until the barbell touches the floor and your chest is again parallel to the ground.

Alternate between the two positions for a complete back workout.

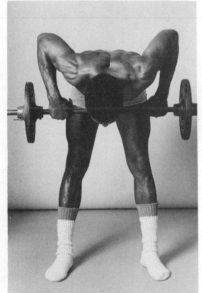

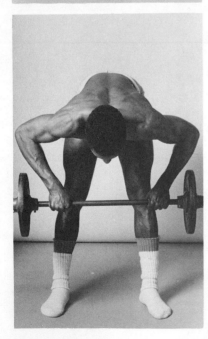

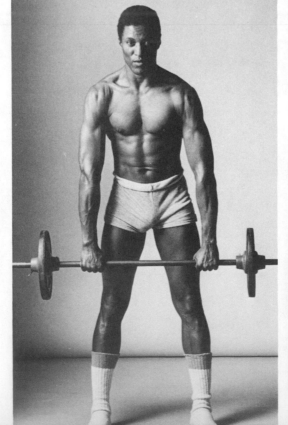

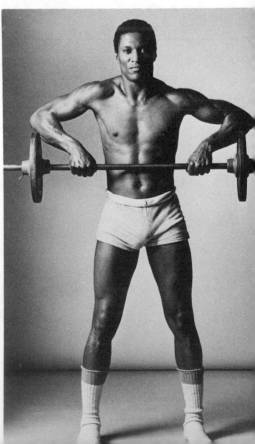

THE DEADLIFT

Position.

Stand before a barbell with your feet spread shoulder width. Squat down deeply, bending completely at your knees, and clasp the barbell, one hand in an overhand grip, the other in an underhand grip for greater stability. Your hands should be a little wider on the bar than the spread of your feet. (Don't load on too much weight too soon. Even though this is the easiest way to lift a sizable amount of weight, it's also easy to strain the back past its limit. Pay particular attention to perfecting your technique for this lift.)

Progression.

Leaning forward with your arms fully extended, initially using the muscle power from your legs, push up with your legs to raise the weight from the floor.

When the barbell is on its way, begin raising your back to a vertical position.

Straighten your legs and your back until you're completely erect.

Shrug back your shoulders, arching your back, and hold your chin up.

With your main strength coming from the legs, not your back, lower the barbell again. Keep looking forward as you squat, bending the knees and trying not to arch your back.

Barely touch the floor with the weight before pushing off with your legs and lifting again.

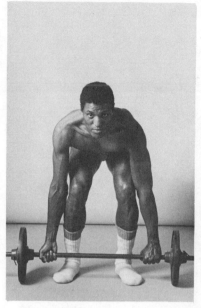

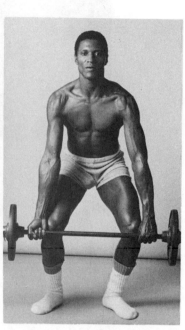

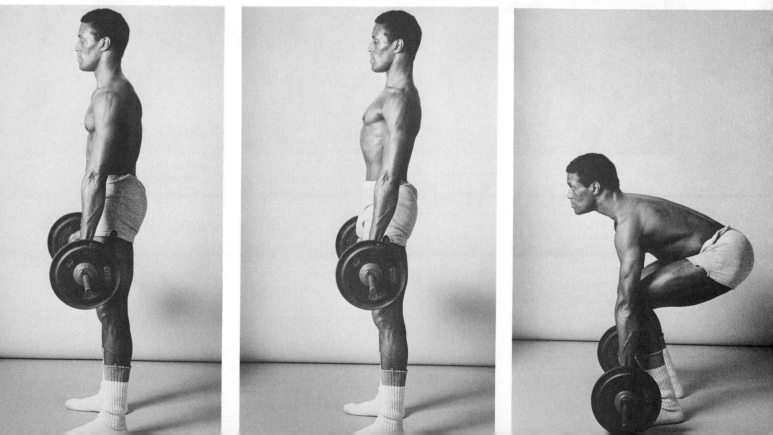

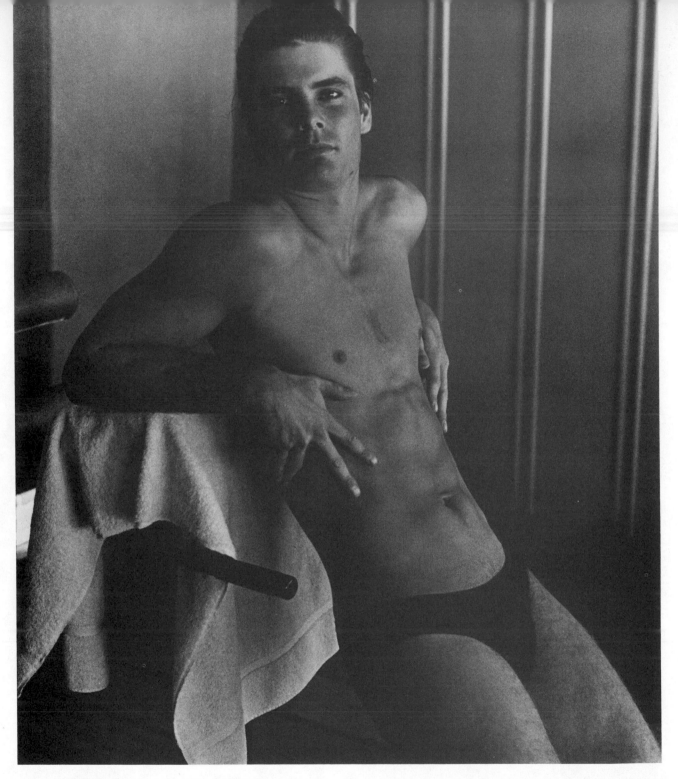

THE WAIST

An hourglass waist is not the goal of your workout. A waist free of love handles and excess flab is. The muscle groups requiring special attention to avoid any spare-tire effect are the intercostals (located at the upper sides of the waist) and the obliques (found at the lower sides of the waist). Also contributing to the waist's appearance are the upper and lower abdominals. These are so important, in fact, they deserve a whole section of exercises of their own.

The Dumb Bend makes a direct attack against love handles. The Seated Twist goes directly for the intercostals and the obliques while helping tighten the lower back. The Bent Twist affects the hips as well as the waist.

THE DUMB BEND

Position.

Holding two dumbbells, stand with your arms slightly spread at your sides and your feet fairly close together.

Progression.

Without bouncing, holding your back straight, lower your right arm until your hand is approximately level with your knee. As you do so, raise your left arm in an arc until that hand is pointing directly at the ceiling.

Bring down your lifted arm, following the same arc, while raising your right shoulder until the two dumbbells are aligned at the starting position.

Repeat on the other side.

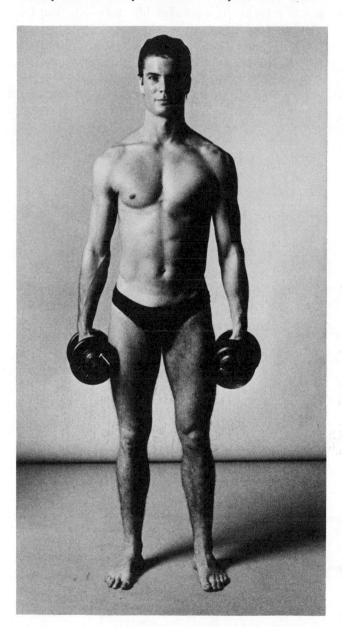

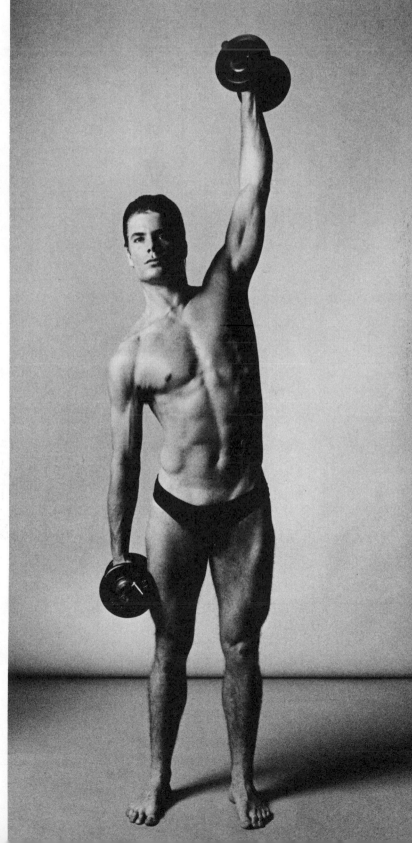

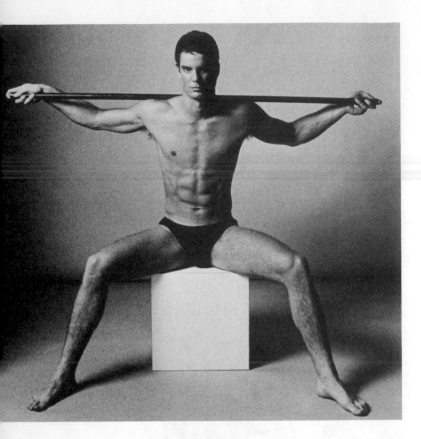

THE SEATED TWIST

Position.

With a pole or the bar of your barbell (minus any weights) resting behind your neck on your shoulders, grasping the bar wide at the ends, straddle the end of the bench (or a cube) with your legs widely spread.

Progression.

Breathing deeply, tense your abdominal muscles as you rotate your right shoulder forward, your left shoulder back.

Reverse your direction, breathing out as you twist your left shoulder forward and your right shoulder back, maintaining tense stomach muscles.

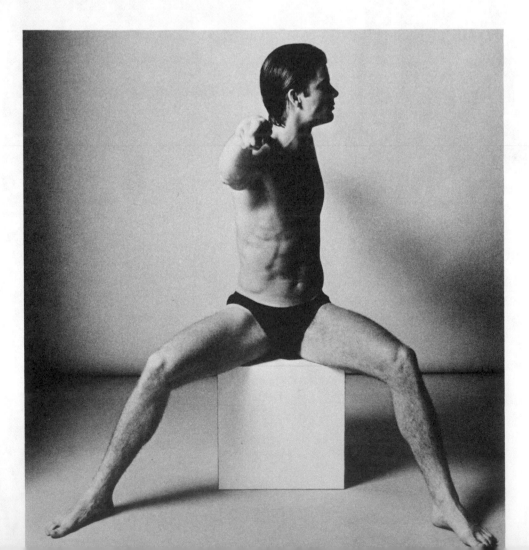

THE BENT TWIST

Position.

Standing with your feet widely spread, rest a pole (or the bar of your barbell) behind your neck on your shoulders, grasping the bar toward each end.

Progression.

Bending at the waist with no arch to your back, keeping it parallel to the floor, with your knees ever so slightly bent, twist at the waist, drawing your left hand down while raising your right arm. Do not move your head or your hips.

Stop rotating the bar just before it reaches the floor in front of your right foot. Keep your gut tensed.

Twisting at the waist in the other direction, reverse the rotation of the bar until the other end reaches the spot in front of your left foot.

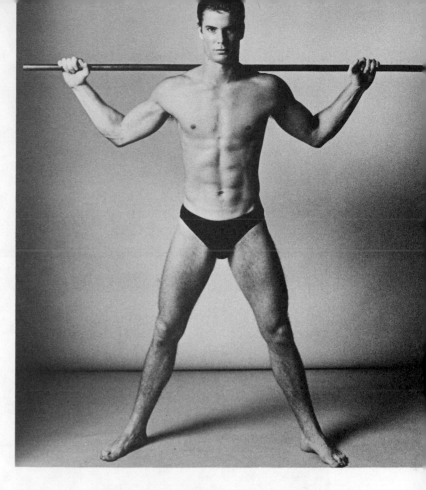

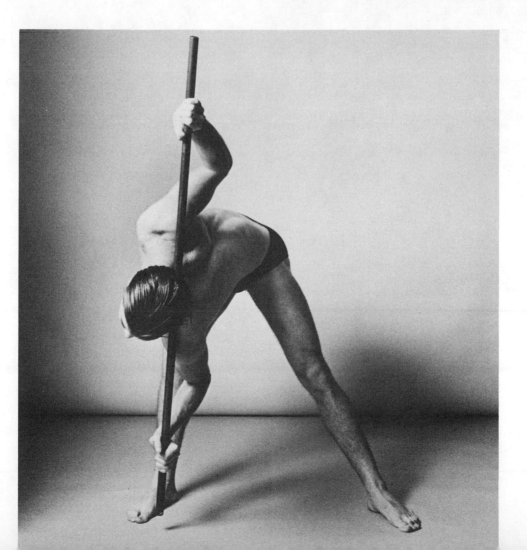

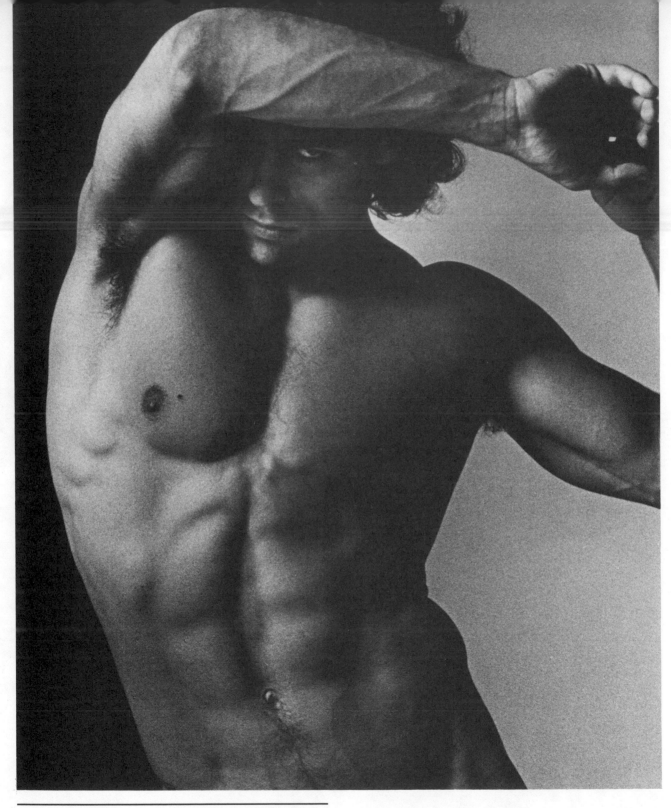

THE ABDOMEN

What more is there to say about abdominal muscles? Only that they demand as much attention as you can give them. It isn't fair that a flat belly is the badge of a great physique, but who said life was fair? For an excellent—not merely fair—ranking, persevere with your abdominal exercises religiously.

Only The Back-Up involves weights, and light ones at that. That's because your abdominal muscles respond more to stretching movements than to weight manipulation. If you like, you can incorporate The Ankle-Up and The Knee-Up in your limbering phase. These exercises are listed here only to reemphasize the point that you can't overlook your abdominals very long without paying a cruel price.

THE ANKLE-UP

Position.

Lie with your back flat on the floor, your hands palm down placed under your buttocks for support. Or, if you prefer, lie down on the bench, with your butt near one end, clasping the side for leverage. Your feet should be together in either case.

Progression.

With your knees barely bent, inhale, then slowly raise your legs (ankles touching) until they form about a 45-degree angle to the floor.

Exhaling, slowly lower your legs, keeping your ankles together and your knees only slightly bent, until your heels are nearly touching the floor (if you're lying on the floor) or until they're parallel to the floor (if you're exercising on a bench).

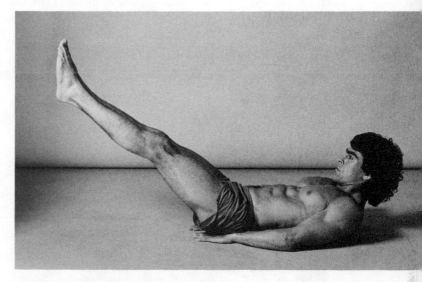

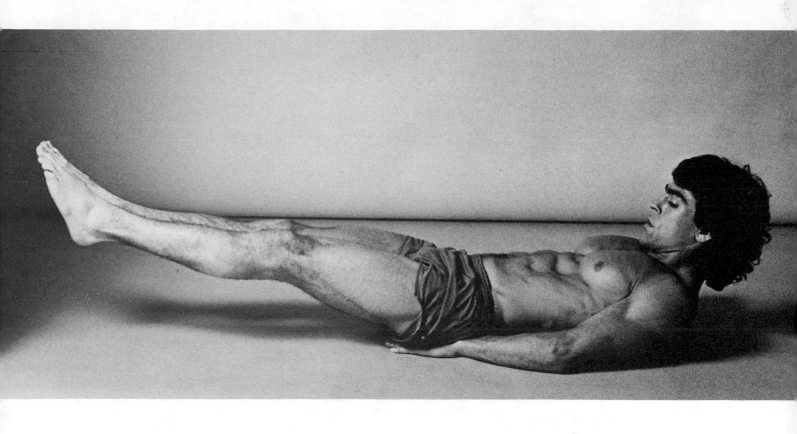

THE KNEE-UP

Position.

Resting on your elbows, lie on the floor with your back slightly raised and your legs straight out in front of you, your heels lifted a few inches off the ground.

Progression.

Leaving your left leg in a stationary position, draw your right knee as close to your forehead as you can.

Extending your right leg back out, at the same time bring your left knee as far as you can toward your forehead. When your right leg is fully extended, keep it straight and a few inches off the floor.

Work your legs back and forth in the same way.

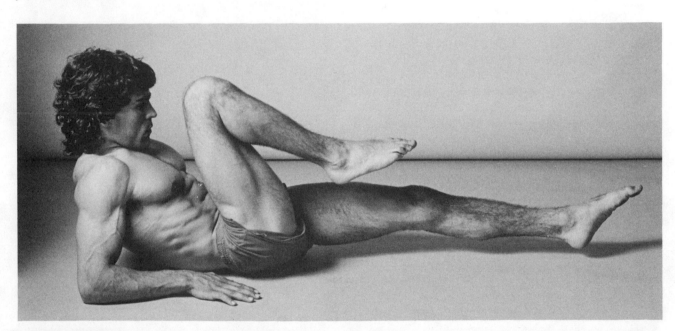

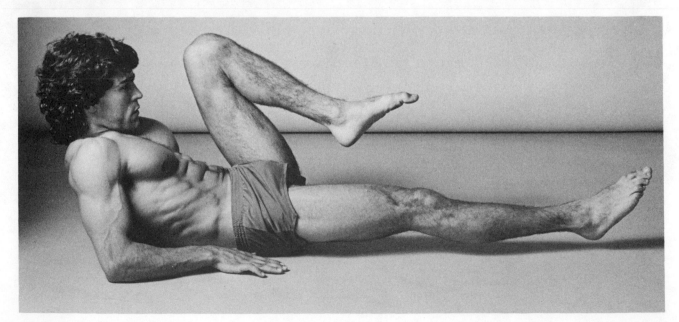

THE BACK-UP

Position.

Wrap a 2½-pound weight in a towel. Lie on your back with your knees bent. Hold the toweled weight in both hands behind your neck. (Don't do this if you have any back problems. Also, do without the weight until your abdominals are quite strong. As you progress, increase the weight.)

Progression.

Without bouncing to gain momentum, with your abdominal muscles tightened, slowly raise your back to an upright position.

Slowly lower yourself again, taking care not to bonk yourself with the weight.

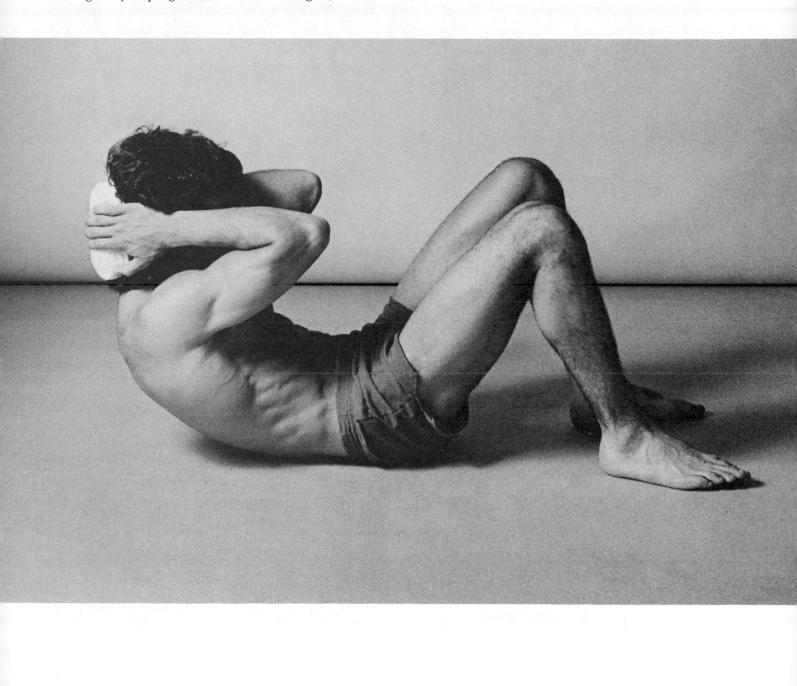

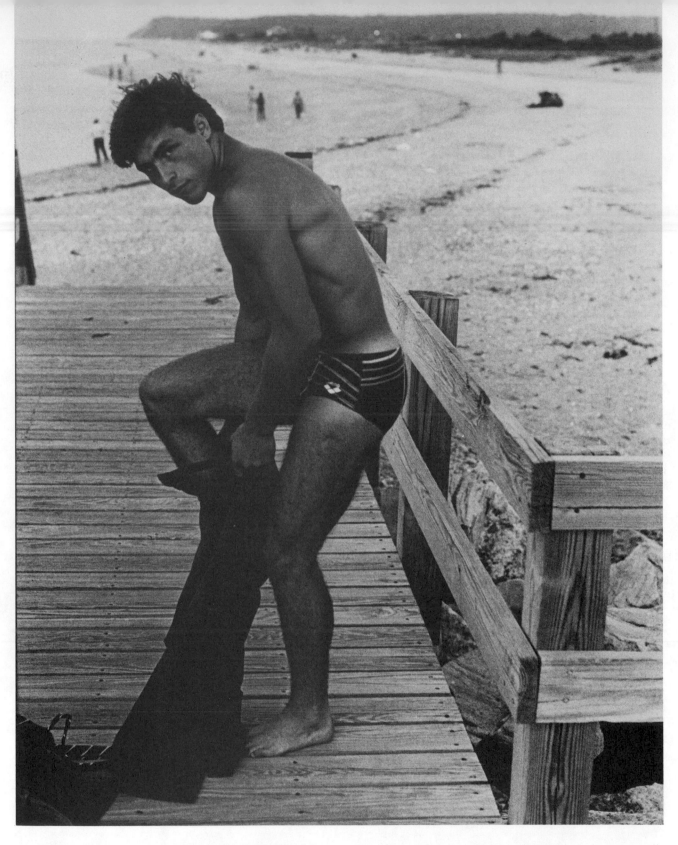

THE BUTTOCKS

Gravity is the grave weapon pulling against your buttocks muscles, and a sagging ass simply doesn't look good. To fight off nature's force, it's smart to shape up these muscles you seldom see; even boxer trunks on the beach can't completely conceal the state of your behind.

Like all the buttocks shapers, The Swing does more than that; it also stimulates your entire body. The Kick is also very helpful in tautening your inner thighs. The Kneel works out thighs and hips too.

THE SWING

Position.

With your feet moderately spread, stand grasping a dumbbell in both hands, raising it straight above your head.

Progression.

Drawing a deep breath, puff up your chest and tense the muscles in your behind.

Breathing out slowly, bend your knees somewhat, lean forward, and swing the weight between your legs, pushing it back past your heels while maintaining a straight position in your arms.

Breathing deeply as you progress so that your chest is fully expanded at the completion, swing the dumbbell back through your legs and lift it in an arc over your head.

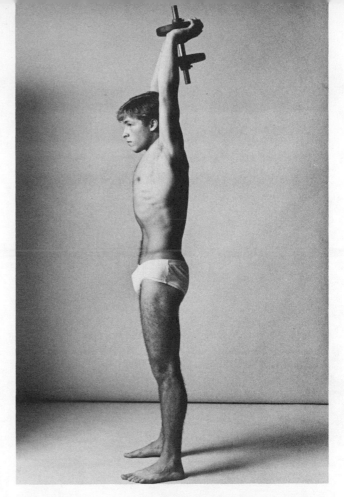

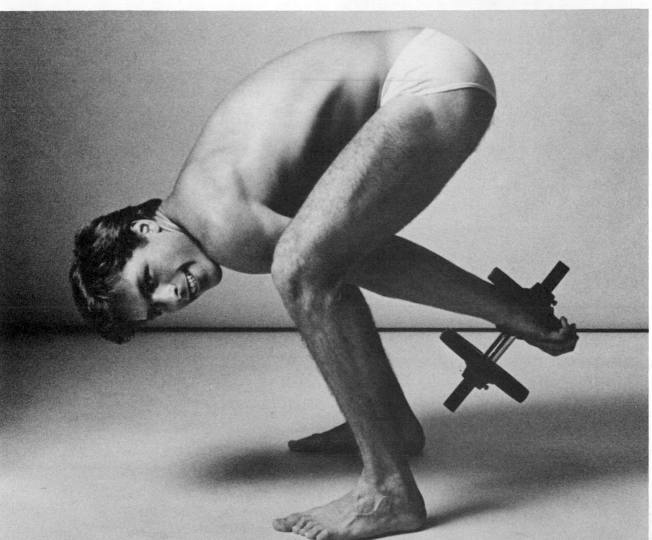

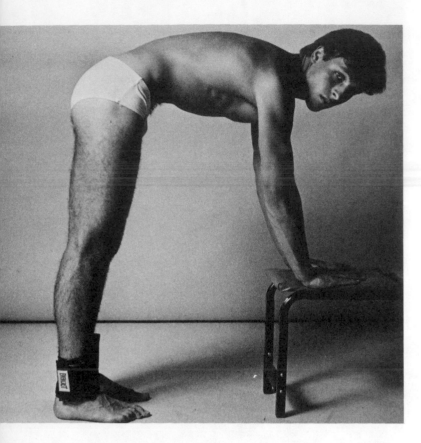

THE KICK

Position.

Wearing ankle weights with your feet nearly together a yard or so away from a bench, bend over and place your palms on top of the bench. Your head should be only a little higher than your hips.

Progression.

Rotating it sideways, raise your right foot behind you to make a continuous straight line (if possible) from your shoulder to your ankle.

Reverse the step until your foot is again on the floor.

Do the same movements with your left leg.

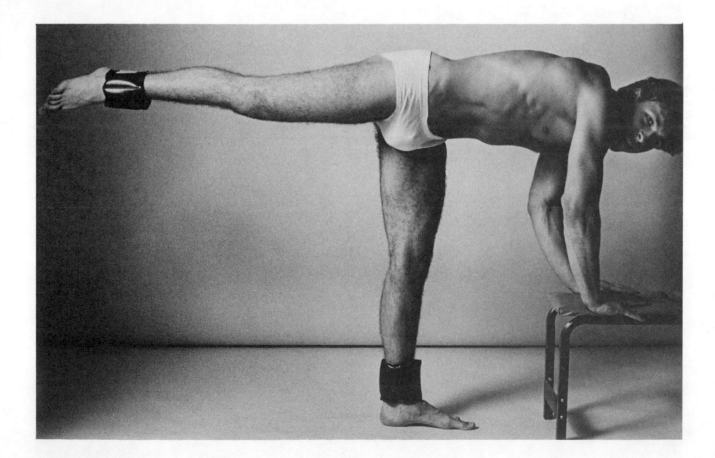

THE KNEEL

Position.

Wearing ankle weights, kneel on the floor on your hands and knees, your back parallel to the floor, with your head looking down.

Progression.

Taking a deep breath, slowly exhale as you raise your right leg behind you and swing it in an arc, pointing it behind you as far as possible.

Inhaling, draw your leg back, careful not to bump your knee against the floor, and tuck your knee as close as you can to your chest while keeping your left leg stationary.

Follow the same procedure with your left leg, keeping butt and gut muscles tight throughout the exercise.

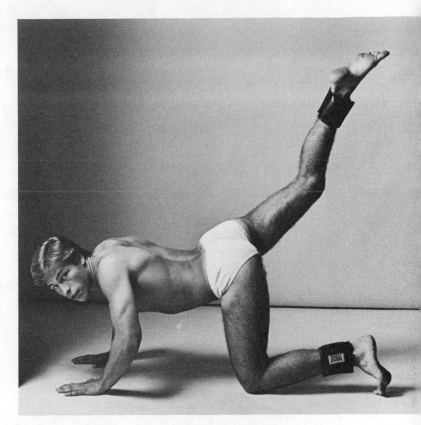

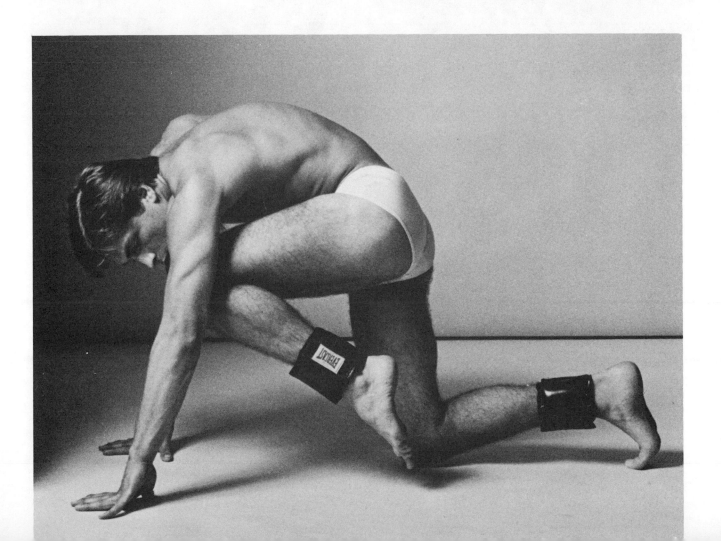

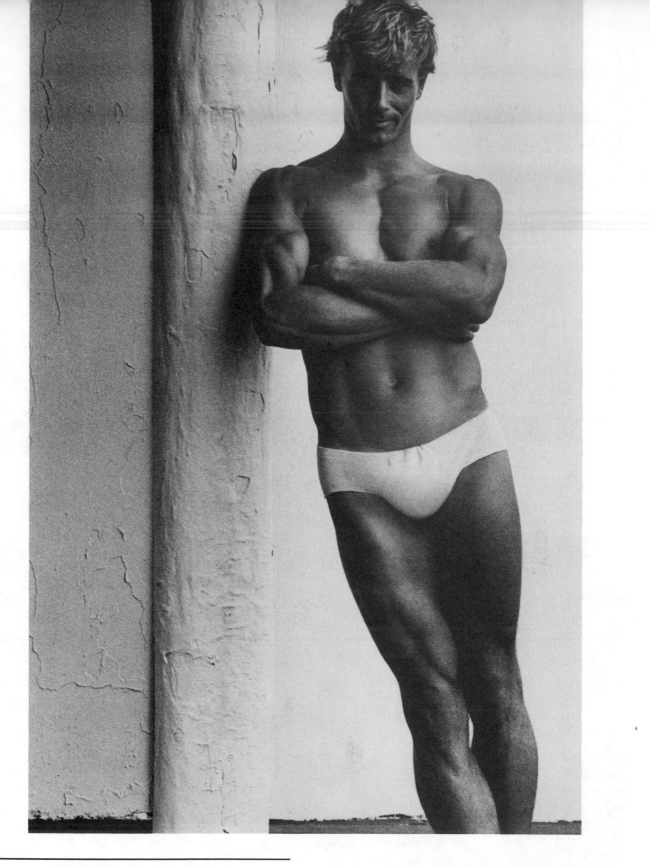

THE LEGS

The leg muscles get residual benefits from most exercises, but it's good to give them some special attention. This is especially needful, in fact, for the calves, since they tend to be obstinately resistant to enlarging.

The Toe-the-Line was developed specifically for calf muscles. The Up-Front Squat works out the thighs thoroughly, as does The Lunge-Up.

THE TOE-THE-LINE

Position.

Using a pole or the bar of a barbell for balance, stand with your feet about a foot apart, toes and balls of your feet on a calf block, heels unsupported.

Progression.

Inhaling, slowly lower your heels as far as possible without touching them to the floor . . . and without tumbling off the block.

Now lift your heels back up and keep raising them until you're standing on your toes, exhaling as you do so. (Raising yourself in this manner, so your heels go straight up with your toes pointed straight ahead, works both sides of the calf.)

Pointing your toes in (to work out the outer calf more completely), lower your heels, then lift them up again.

Standing on the ball of your right foot, bend your knee and raise your left foot.

Inhaling, raise your right heel until you're standing on your toes.

Exhaling, slowly lower your heel as far as possible before lifting again.

Repeat the procedure while standing on the ball of your left foot with your right knee bent. (One-legged raises give the entire calf an extra-good workout.)

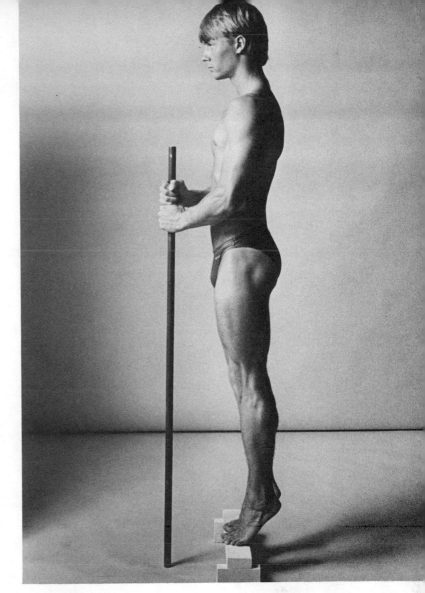

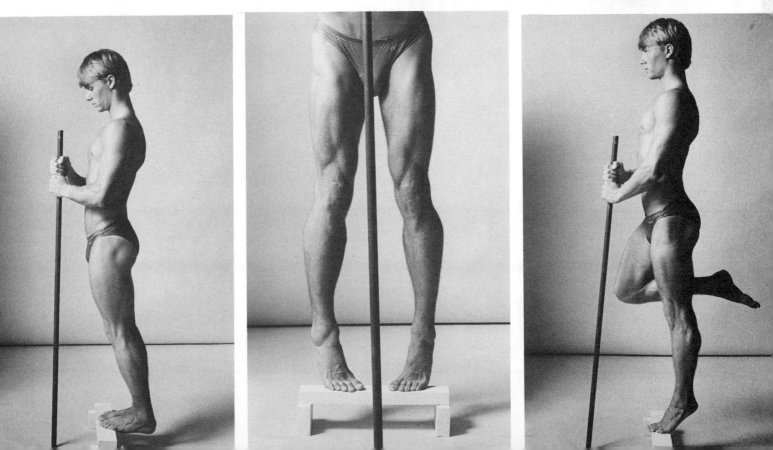

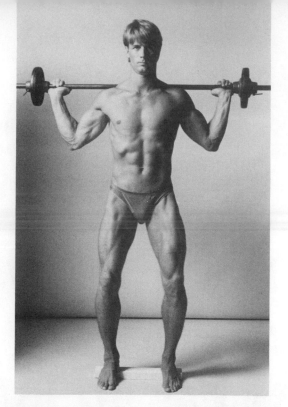

THE UP-FRONT SQUAT

Position.

Standing with your heels on a low block, feet about a foot apart, rest a barbell (held in the overhand grip) with less weight than usual on your shoulders.

Progression.

Inhale, your chin level and your eyes straight ahead; bend your knees and slowly lower yourself, keeping your back straight, until your thighs are parallel to the floor.

Slowly raise yourself to the original position and exhale.

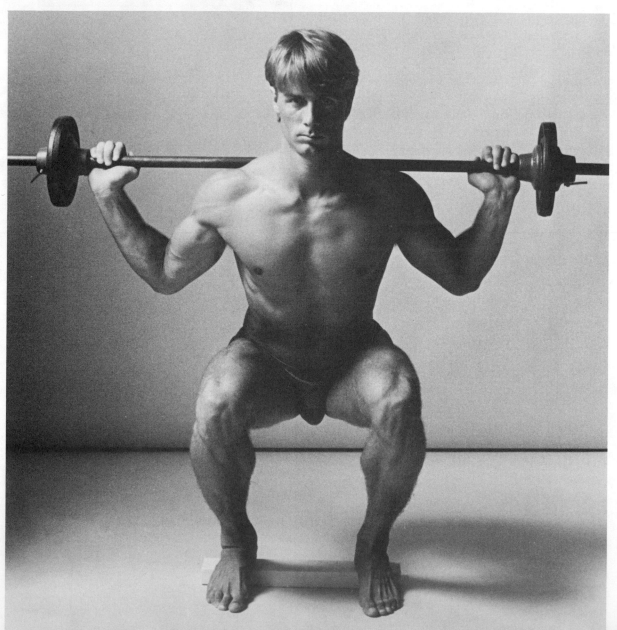

THE LUNGE-UP

Position.

With a dumbbell in each hand, put your right foot on a bench and extend your left foot far behind you until you're leaning on your toes.

Progression.

Inhaling, move your raised knee forward, bending as you proceed, until your weight is primarily on the right foot and your left leg is fully stretched. Keep your back straight.

Exhaling, push with your right leg until you've raised yourself to the original position.

Repeat with the other leg.

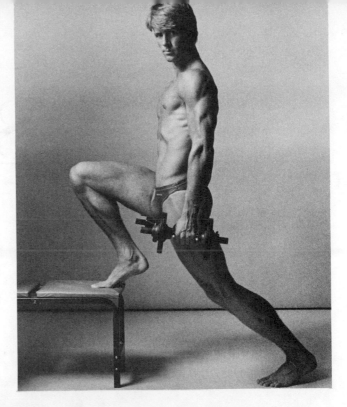

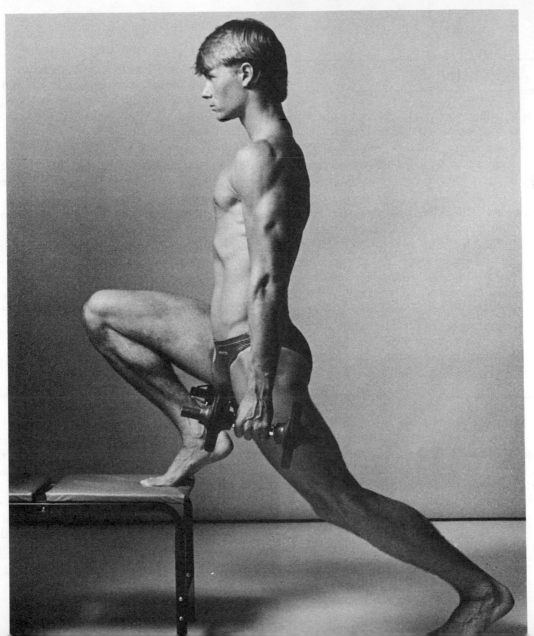

CHAPTER 8

NEW MATH

PLUS AND MINUS

Think back to when you started reading this book. Remember taking some elementary tests to help you get a fix on your general level of fitness? (If you didn't take them, flip back to Chapter 1 and go through them now.) Recall how you checked your pulse to get a rough idea of the maximum heart rate you should never exceed when working out? (If you don't, the formula was subtracting your age from 200.) Well, it's time for some refinement.

It only stands to reason that someone whose cardiovascular system and muscular development are both in tip-top shape is able to work out more vigorously than another person who's been going to seed for year upon year. The former could probably do most of the exercises described in the last four chapters with relative ease, while the latter could probably do few of them without severe twinges. The big question is: Where do you fit in? Are you fit? going to seed? or somewhere in between?

Since you've undergone the tests, you already have an approximate notion of the shape you're in. With that partial knowledge, you can get more specific about your exercise needs and safeguards.

In an attempt to raise the fitness level of its employees, the Xerox Corporation created a series of exercises called the Xerox Health Management Program. Basically geared toward aerobics, the program is more rudimentary than the routines outlined in this chapter, but it includes a precise (and admittedly somewhat complicated) way to measure how intensely you are exercising. (This measurement also informs you if you're exercising *too* intensely.)

The guidelines are based on the "training heartbeat"—the pulse rate to which you must rise to receive aerobic conditioning without exercising too strenuously for your own good.

Here is the formula: 220 (the absolute maximum your heart can beat and still pump blood to the body), minus your age, minus your resting heartbeat, times 60 percent if you're in poor or only fair condition (times 70 percent if you're in average condition, or times 80 percent if you're in good or excellent condition), plus your resting heartbeat.

Whew!

Say you're thirty, in average condition, and your resting heartbeat is 70. Subtracting 30 (your age) from 220 (maximum heartbeat), you get 190. Subtracting 70 (resting heartbeat), you get 120. Multiplying by .7 (because you're in average condition), the subtotal is 84. Adding 70 (resting heartbeat again), you arrive at 154—your "training heartbeat," the pulse rate you safely want to rise to but not exceed during the height of your workout. *Right now.*

After you've improved your overall fitness to excellent (still operating on the hypothesis that you're thirty), your training heartbeat can—and, for you to maintain that level of excellence, *should*—go as

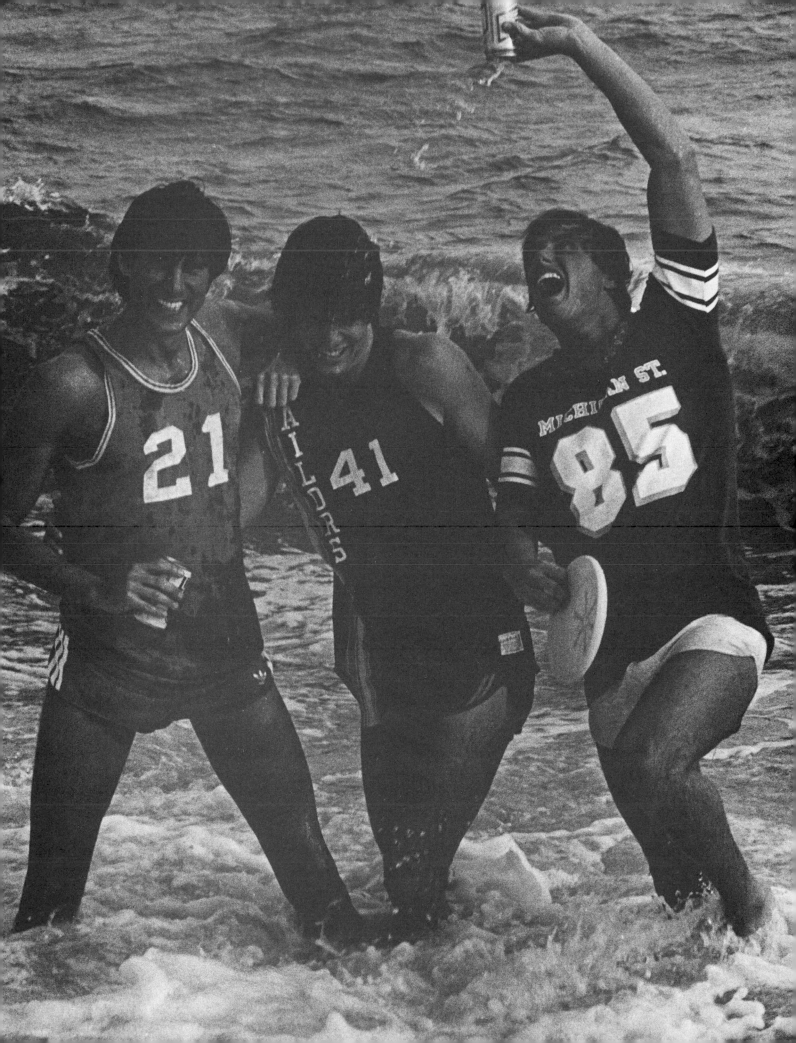

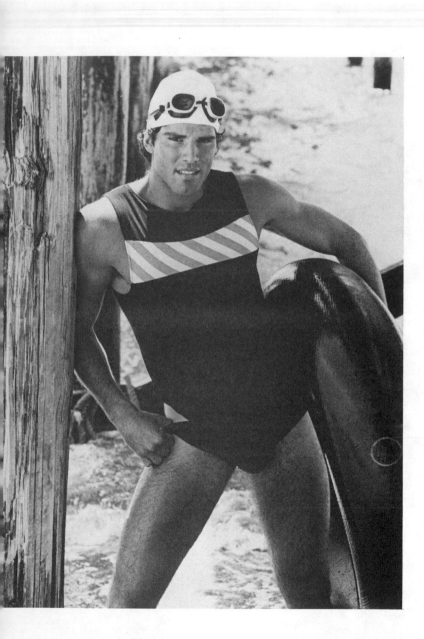

high as 166 heartbeats per minute. The formula offers the proof: Subtracting the age 30 from 220, then subtracting the resting heartbeat of 70, you still arrive at 120. But now you multiply by .8 (representing excellent physical condition), and you get a subtotal of 96. Adding the resting heartbeat again, the sum is 166 for the desired training heartbeat. That means you've increased your work capacity by 12 heartbeats per minute. Not bad at all.

Of course, if you work out exceedingly well, you will eventually lower your resting heartbeat, removing some strain from your heart. Although this theoretically lowers your training heartbeat during exercise, the practical consequence is still a gain, since the heart is getting more out of every pump at less risk.

Continuing to hypothesize you're thirty with a resting heartbeat of 70 but not yet at your excellent physical prime, your training heartbeat will be under 166. If you're in poor condition, it will be 150. If you're forty and in average shape, it will be 144. If you're forty-five and have gone to pot, it will be 141. Conversely, at a shaped-up forty-five, your training heartbeat will be 153—the same training heartbeat as for a twenty-five-year-old in poor condition!

The training heartbeat is a more sophisticated reference point than simply knowing your maximum heartbeat. After all, there's no reason to force your heart to literally pound itself if you can improve your fitness with less strain and stress. So don't ever think you'll be shaping up faster if you work out too hard. You won't. And you might not be around to testify to your dangerous folly.

Naturally enough, you do not plow into exercising at your training heartbeat. While you're warming up, your pulse should be much nearer your resting heartbeat. Your pulse during the limbering phase should be between the two. Even when you're involved in progressive resistance, your pulse rate should not be at the maximum rate consistently. Only during aerobic activity do you purposefully sustain the rigors of the training heartbeat. For optimum benefit, your goal is to work out nonstop at this pulse level for twenty to thirty minutes every other day. If your heartbeat ever gets higher, slow down. If your heartbeat remains too high at a decelerated pace, rest awhile.

Even though the training heartbeat is fundamentally a gauge for aerobic activities, it's helpful in determining your physical status and progress. If you've judged yourself to be in average shape but if your pulse is pumping at the training heartbeat pace while you're warming up or limbering, you're not as shaped-up as you think. On the other hand, even though you've decided you're in poor shape and are consequently working out on the light side, if your pulse doesn't rise to the training heartbeat pitch during maintenance exercise, you're in better condition than you think and you should be pushing yourself harder by exercising faster. If you can't stand the thought of stepping up your pace, then you'll have to exercise much, much longer to receive any training effect. For example, when you're working at only 20-percent capacity, to get the same cardiovascular gain as you would when exercising at 60 percent of your maximum heartbeat for ten minutes, you must work out for three hours! Wouldn't you rather speed it up instead? But not prematurely, of course.

STAGE DOORS

Okay, now that you've rated yourself as being in poor, average, or excellent condition, how does this assessment affect your workouts? Theoretically, your fitness rating places you in one of the following workout levels: The Rookie Stage—for beginners, particularly anyone over thirty who hasn't exercised regularly or only now and again on weekends for most of his adult life; The Player Stage—for fellows who have been active enough to keep in decent shape but who haven't been truly systematic about their exercise; and The Pro Stage—for guys already in excellent shape, regardless of how they fell into this state of grace.

However, the results of your tests may not work out that neatly. It may be that you've been running regularly and qualify for The Pro Stage in maintenance exercises, but your flexibility may be way down below par, so you'll be slotted in The Rookie Stage for limbering. Similarly, maybe you've never lifted weights but you could be strong enough to pump along at The Player Stage. Your inexperience with weight-lifting technique would place you in The Rookie Stage until familiarity with weights allows you to jump to The Player Stage.

If you're a mixed qualifier, look on the bright side: Because your fitness level is not uniformly poor, odds are you'll improve rapidly in those areas where you're presently lacking. Your ascent to

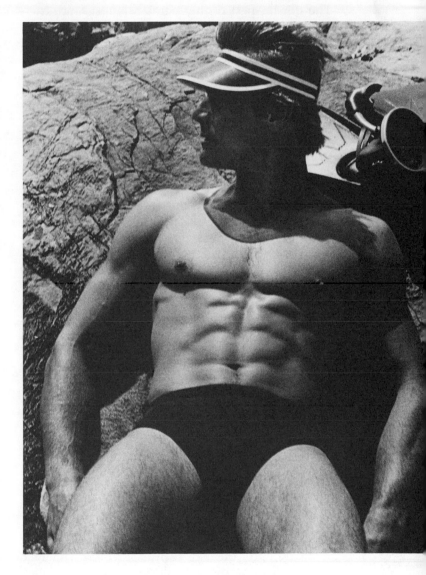

overall excellence won't be a steep climb, particularly if your aerobic capability is good.

The exercise plan that follows is designed to work out every part of your body to achieve several significant ends. The first is cardiovascular fitness. Regardless of your body type, this is always the primary goal. Second, the program gives high priority to developing a flexible, supple body through stretching. In terms of longevity, flexibility is not as crucial as cardiovascular fitness, but it is highly desirable for both how you look and how you feel. The third aspect of the regimen is resistance exercise. This is the area where you will have the major input in modification, depending upon your goals. As long as you conscientiously apply yourself to aerobic and limbering activities, you will have a healthy, well-functioning body. But to alter muscular dimensions—which may or may not be your goal—you must rely on resistance exercises.

Although this may be surprising to you, if your principal aim is to tone your body while improving your cardiovascular fitness and your flexibility, you will follow the same general program regardless whether you have a Burly, Sinewy, or Stringy frame. How so? Because all you're asking of yourself is to make up for any current lack in fitness. The same is true if you want to build up your musculature only to a minor degree. Why? Because you will be working on *every* body part for *overall* muscular improvement. Only when you're attempting a major overhaul of your physique, with specific body areas requiring intensive attention and focus, will your regimen differ dramatically from someone else's. In essence, the more precise you make your goals, the more individual attention you must give to tailoring your workouts to attain those goals.

THE ROOKIE STAGE

This is the most disheartening stage, because initially the terrain looks endless. Don't you believe it. Even though you may feel as if you're crawling, you're covering distance all the same. Remember, you're only measuring your own progress. And if you need any additional reassurance, think about this: Even professional body builders are no further ahead than you, because they too are constantly, ceaselessly striving to better their physiques. Whether you're a Rookie or a Pro, working out is never anything more than making the best of *you*.

Now for the various segments of your workout.

TUNING EXERCISES

Never skimp on the time given to warming up. You should allow *a full eight to ten minutes* for tuning up. If you're no longer a youngster and have been sedentary for some time, allocate even more time if you possibly can as a precaution. Also, if you're in pretty poor shape you probably won't be able to execute all of these warm-ups, and you definitely won't be able to do all the limbering exercises that follow. If you go about warming up at a leisurely and extended pace, you'll be improving your overall body condition without too many jerks and jolts. You'll purposefully avoid operating full-steam at your training heartbeat, so the more time you can give yourself for *slowly* warming up, the better. Thankfully, you have a whole lifetime ahead of you in which to get going faster and harder. But if you can't be that casual, eight to ten minutes of *moderate* tune-up activity will do you no harm and lots of good.

At this stage, at least try to do all the tuning exercises, but don't push too hard to complete those beyond your abilities. For now, you should attempt to execute all of them in one fashion or another a minimum of three times within ten minutes. Rest when you feel like it, but preferably not for more than half a minute each slow-down. If you start feeling breathless, lessen your output even further. Check your pulse every three or four minutes (less often, of course, after you've been exercising regularly) to make certain you are nowhere near your training heartbeat. If you start feeling dizzy, cease. Nausea and any pain in the chest are also stop signs.

Don't move past the tuning stage if you can't get through it without a heaving chest. If you're having that much difficulty, spend lots of time walking between exercise sessions. Only when you can comfortably get through a warm-up without undue breathlessness or dizziness should you expand your workout.

On the other hand, assuming your only difficulty while tuning up is flawless execution and you're not experiencing any great physical discomfort after warming up, move on.

To progress to The Player Stage, you should be doing all the warm-ups at least five times each within a ten-minute span.

LIMBERING EXERCISES

Don't skimp on limbering either. Allow *a minimum of fifteen minutes*, more if you've got the time and inclination, but don't exceed half an hour. If

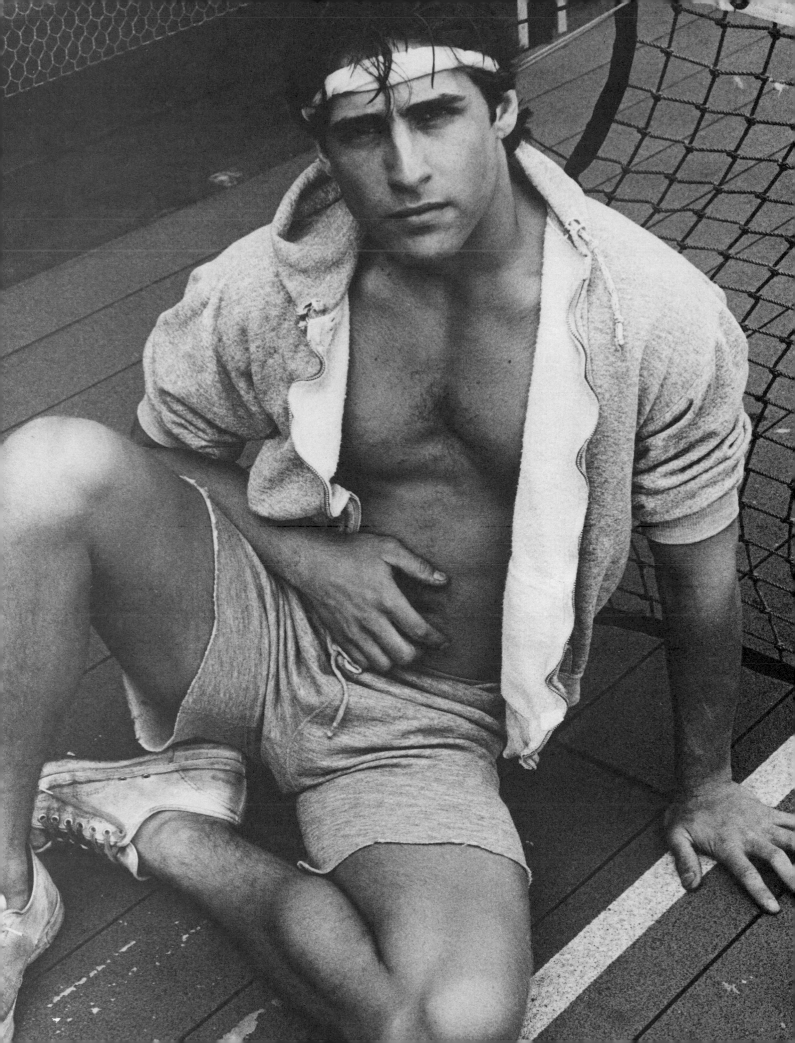

you go that long, lace the session with several rest periods. Needless to say, pain signifies reckless abandon.

Proceed with the same caution you exercised while warming up. Ideally you should do each of these stretches at least three times. (In those instances when you're told to exercise on alternate sides—as in The "Elbow-in-the Ear" on page 63, for example—three times means three times on each side. In exercises incorporating several steps—such as The Straddle Stretch on page 70—you must execute all the steps to complete the exercise once, so three times means executing the complete exercise three times.) Do what you can as fully and accurately as possible, giving three good efforts, then move on to the next exercise. If you finish all your sets before the fifteen minutes are up, start over and do every exercise one more time in sequence until your time is up.

If you don't finish all the stretches within fifteen minutes and you're not feeling bushed, *slowly* continue until you've finished or until your body warns you to quit. Make sure you never exceed your training heartbeat. Preferably, you should remain below it. At first, measure your pulse every three minutes or so until your intuition can take over.

Stay at this level for a few weeks, then increase your sets to four reps each. A couple of weeks later, increase the number of reps to five. *You cannot advance to The Player Stage until you can do one set of five reps of all the stretches fairly easily (if not perfectly) within fifteen minutes,* so each day try a little harder. But not if you notice any danger signals.

If you ever feel very tired after limbering, rest for a few minutes to regroup. Really pooped? Then call it a day. If your pulse is over 120 five minutes after quitting, you've been too rough and tough on yourself. Ten minutes after halting, if your pulse is over 100, that's no good either. (These time periods and pulse rates are applicable to all types of exercises, not just limbering.) And if you're still short of breath ten minutes after stopping a workout, you need to treat yourself more kindly and work out more slowly.

MAINTENANCE EXERCISES

Because of the intense way they tax our cardiovascular system, you must be very careful with your aerobics when starting out. If your condition is very poor, hold off for a couple of weeks before even initiating maintenance exercises. Simply warming up and stretching—and lots of walking—will help prepare you for the necessary rigors of aerobics.

You can postpone them, but not indefinitely. They're your most important fitness tools.

When you do start, if at all possible, try to afford yourself a large chunk of time. If you could jog quite slowly for half an hour with a heartbeat of 135 at the beginning operations of The Rookie Stage, for example, that would be preferable to taking on ten minutes of aerobics at a heartbeat of 150, and the cardiovascular benefit would be comparable. If you've time on your hands, take the slower aerobic path for a while. Not because it would be hazardous to raise your heartbeat to 150, but because it would be a little safer not going above 135 the first or second time out.

If you don't have the luxury of time, however, start out with any maintenance exercise you like. Boxing (page 95) is good for the real novice. Begin for about a minute at or slightly below your training heartbeat, then walk or stretch to rest for thirty seconds before stepping up your pace with the same or another aerobic exercise performed at or slightly below your training heartbeat. Severely reduce your activity for thirty seconds again. Get livelier for another minute. Go on and almost off like this for a total of ten minutes your first time out. Even if you feel up to doing much more much longer, don't.

Gradually increase your aerobic activity and decrease your at-rest intervals. Check your heartbeat every three minutes until you've developed a sense for the status of your pulse. Do not exceed your desired training heartbeat. Always watch out for yourself. Don't ignore danger signals.

When you can comfortably maintain fifteen minutes of aerobic activity at your stipulated training heartbeat after your limbering routine, you will be in much better shape, ready to graduate to The Player Stage. Of course, you'll probably also want to partake of progressive-resistance routines even as a Rookie.

BUILDING EXERCISES

As you're well aware, lifting weights doesn't qualify as an aerobic activity. But resistance exercises put a strain—often a great strain—on the heart nonetheless, since they are fueled by bursts of energy. For that reason, if you're a Rookie, you should start building your aerobic fitness before undertaking weights. On the other hand, you needn't possess the aerobic capabilities of a marathon man before you start building muscle mass. Just make certain that you can stretch reasonably well and can perform aerobics for fifteen minutes comfortably before tackling resistance exercises.

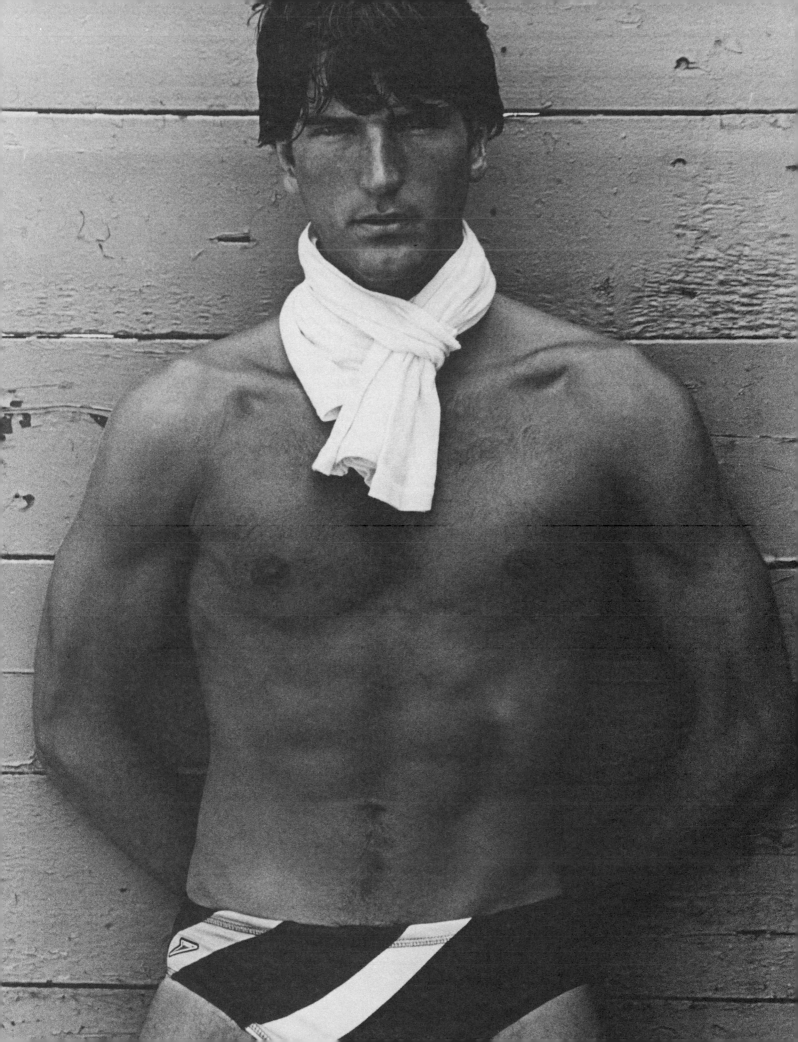

Be just as slow when embarking on your building phase as you were initiating aerobics. At first, simply aim for completing as many of the exercises as you can once, using what might seem excessively light weights, so that you feel hardly any strain at all, *within a ten-minute building session.*

On your next day of resistance routines, if you didn't complete the full circuit of exercises your first day out, start off where you finished the last time, still using very light weights.

Work very slowly in this manner for a few weeks to get the feel for both the weights and the movements, tagging on an extra minute each few days until you're working out for fifteen minutes. Don't champ at the bit with impatience. If you think you're wasting endless amounts of time, just think how long it took you to get into the poor condition that dictates your cautious pacing now.

Once you've reached the fifteen-minute exercise level, if you're still using relatively light weights—and you *should* still be using them—you shouldn't be having any difficulty getting through all twenty-nine building exercises once. So increase the weights a little (five pounds more should be about right) and set out to do each of the exercises twice. Quicken your pace, but you'll still need a little more time than fifteen minutes—about twenty minutes should do.

In truth, you're not adding bulging muscles while proceeding in this nonstressful fashion. Light weights only tone muscles; heavy ones build bigger muscles. But rehearsal time to become more familiar with weight-lifting technique is always time well spent. And your body *is* being gently conditioned.

Keep adding a minute or two to your sessions, and slowly increase the amount of weight you're lifting. You'll probably discover you can lift more weight in some exercises, not so much in others, as your body most likely isn't uniformly strong. The weaker areas are the spots you should spend more time—and more exercise—developing. Rest whenever you need to.

Once you're up to *thirty-minute building workouts,* get serious. Strive to complete each exercise three times within that time span, utilizing enough weight so you feel thoroughly tired—but not spent—when you're through.

At that point, it will be time to develop new strategies.

You've been doing a total of three different exercises (in the case of your arms, five) for each part of your body in order to effect overall improvement when easing into the building routine. Variety is a good way to keep all your muscles exercised, but high numbers of repetitions of particular exercises are also desirable. To increase the number of reps per set without adding time to your exercise session, you must reduce the number of exercises while increasing the intensity of effort you put into those you'll be doing.

The best way to do this is to choose only one exercise from each group (excepting arms and legs, where you'll choose two) and set a goal of ten reps per set for each individual exercise, varying the exercises chosen from each group from one workout to the next. (To review four different schedules for four days of resistance workouts, refer to the chart on the opposite page.)

Proceed this way for about a month, gradually adding more weight. Also, decide on any body area you particularly want to work out during a session and instead of doing one set of ten reps, do two sets of eight reps each on that particular day.

Rest when you have to, but avoid taking breaks in the middle of sets, since the benefit stems principally from the repetitive nature of the movements. Establish a rhythm to your sessions. Do one set, then catch your breath for ten or twenty seconds by improvising a gentle stretch for the muscles you've just worked out. (Lacking in improvisational talent? Then do a warm-up or a limbering movement at a decidedly leisurely pace.) Every couple of sets you might—in fact, probably will—need a little more rest, so simply amble about until your breath and heartbeat are close to normal again. Don't allow your heartbeat to remain too long at its training level in between sets. If you require more time at this point to get your heartbeat down, by all means take it.

When you've reached this level, pat yourself on the back. Think back to when your major accomplishment was just getting through all the exercises once with puny weights in one session. Now you're doing all the exercises at least ten times every three sessions, and you're lifting heavier weights to boot. Good for you, fella.

Your reward? Step right up to The Player Stage.

COOLING EXERCISES

At this level, you probably won't be able to manage the cool-downs as described, so don't try for perfect performance. If you put too much effort into them, you'll be defeating the whole purpose. Spend *five to eight minutes cooling down,* casually going through the motions as far as you comfortably can. If you prefer, slowly walk down your heartbeat until you're breathing normally. You don't need to master the intricacies of cool-down movements to elevate yourself to The Player Stage.

INTENSITY ROUTINES

This chart specifies the building exercises as they are to be performed during the resistance phase at the conclusion of The Rookie Stage—one set of ten reps of each exercise within thirty-minute workouts as designated by days. How quickly you accelerate to this level will depend upon your fitness and familiarity with weight training. To chart your individual course safely and wisely, use the following recommendations—formulated for a male in poor condition with no background in lifting weights—as a guideline for general progress:

• For the first several weeks, do all the exercises *once* in *ten* minutes.

• For the next several weeks, do all the exercises *twice* in *twenty* minutes with heavier weights.

• Over the next several weeks, do all the exercises *three times* in *thirty minutes* with still heavier weights.

• Initiate Intensity Routines. (If you wish to work out a particular area more intensively, occasionally exercise it for two sets of eight reps each, resting a minute or so between sets.)

EXERCISES	DAY 1	DAY 2	DAY 3	DAY 4
NECK				
The Weighted Shrug, p. 107	X	—	—	X
The Lift-and-Shrug, p. 108	—	X	—	—
The Row-Up, p. 109	—	—	X	—
SHOULDERS				
The Dip, p. 111	X	—	—	—
The Press-Back, p. 112	—	X	—	X
The Dumb Lat, p. 113	—	—	X	—
ARMS				
The Curl III, p. 117	X	X	X	X
The Extension I, p. 118	X	—	X	—
The Extension II, p. 119	—	X	—	X
CHEST				
The Push-Off, p. 121	X	—	—	—
The Dumb Fly, p. 122	—	X	—	—
The Dumb Over, p. 123	—	—	X	X
BACK				
The Dumb Row, p. 125	—	X	—	—
The Row-Down, p. 126	X	—	—	X
The Deadlift, p. 127	—	—	X	—
WAIST				
The Dumb Bend, p. 129	X	—	—	—
The Seated Twist, p. 130	—	X	—	X
The Bent Twist, p. 131	—	—	X	—
ABDOMEN				
The Ankle-Up, p. 133	X	—	—	—
The Knee-Up, p. 134	—	X	—	—
The Back-Up, p. 135	—	—	X	X
BUTTOCKS				
The Swing, p. 137	X	—	—	X
The Kick, p. 138	—	X	—	—
The Kneel, p. 139	—	—	X	—
LEGS				
The Toe-the-Line, p. 141	X	X	X	X
The Up-Front Squat, p. 142	X	—	X	—
The Lunge-Up, p. 143	—	X	—	X

SUMMARY

Regardless of body type, the regimens are virtually the same at The Rookie Stage, since you must condition your body before exerting more pressure and before effecting sizable changes in your contours.

EVERY DAY

Tuning Exercises

For the first two to three weeks, allow eight minutes of tune-up activity.

For the next two to three weeks, gradually increase your pace within nine-minute sessions.

Over the following two to three weeks, work up to ten minutes of tune-ups.

Immediately after tuning up, go into your daily limbering phase.

Limbering Exercises

Start out with fifteen minutes of *slow* stretching.

Continue doing fifteen minutes of stretching, gradually increasing the number of reps as time progresses until you have completed The Rookie Stage.

Your daily limbering phase is followed by alternating days of aerobic and resistance exercises.

Cooling Exercises

Always be sure to cool off sufficiently, allowing a minimum of five minutes.

EVERY OTHER DAY

Maintenance Exercises

For the first two to six weeks, depending upon your cardiovascular health, spend ten minutes on stop-and-start aerobics on those days you are *not* doing any resistance exercises. Slowly eliminate the rest periods.

(As is now obvious, your rate of acceleration from stage to stage will differ according to the type of activity. You must proceed more slowly with maintenance exercises than with tuning up, for example, because it's much more possible to harm yourself if you push too strenuously into aerobics. If you overdo on tuning up, the worst that can happen is getting a stiff or strained muscle. Reckless aerobics could cause cardiac arrest.)

During the next four to six weeks, gradually move up to twelve minutes of sustained aerobics.

Over the following four to six weeks, increase your nonstop aerobic activity to fifteen minutes in each every-other-day session.

Building Exercises

These sessions may vary, depending upon your decision about the physique you plan to attain.

If you've definitely decided you don't want to lift weights, don't. In their stead, you could substitute aerobics, although doing so isn't necessary.

If you've decided to tone your muscles by lifting moderate weights, slowly increase the duration of your sessions from ten to fourteen minutes during the first two to three weeks.

For the next two to four weeks, gradually increase the length of your sessions to twenty minutes.

Over the following four to eight weeks, gradually work up to thirty minutes of building exercises every other day.

This is the general program for The Rookie Stage. By the time you finish your tenure as a Rookie, you will be exercising approximately forty-five to sixty minutes a day. Now is the time to consider what effect your genetic body type and the particular body configuration you're seeking will have upon the general program.

THE BURLY BODY

With endomorphy spelled out in your genes, you know that it's unreasonable to aspire to a long and lithe frame. Don't knock your head against the wall with unrealistic expectations.

At this exercise level, *dedication* must be your by-word. Pay particular attention to cardiovascular activities and food consumption. Twisting (page 96) might be more fun, but a rigorous session of Fancy Stepping (page 101) is a more physically profitable maintenance exercise for someone with your inbred propensity toward flab.

If a heavily muscled body is not your goal, use light weights to tone your body. On the other hand, to achieve strong muscle definition, you must concentrate on working out with increasingly heavy weights. Large doses of aerobic *and* resistance labor are essential. But limbering movements can't be ignored, for without them your body will appear—and most likely will remain—uncoordinated.

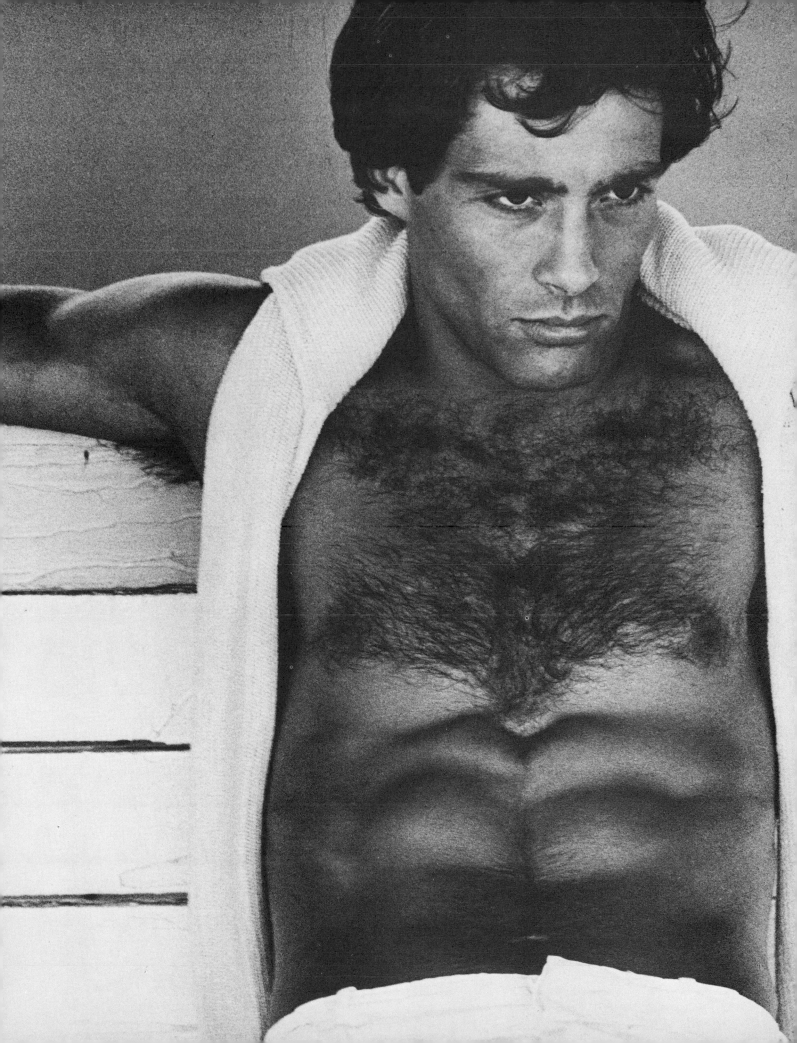

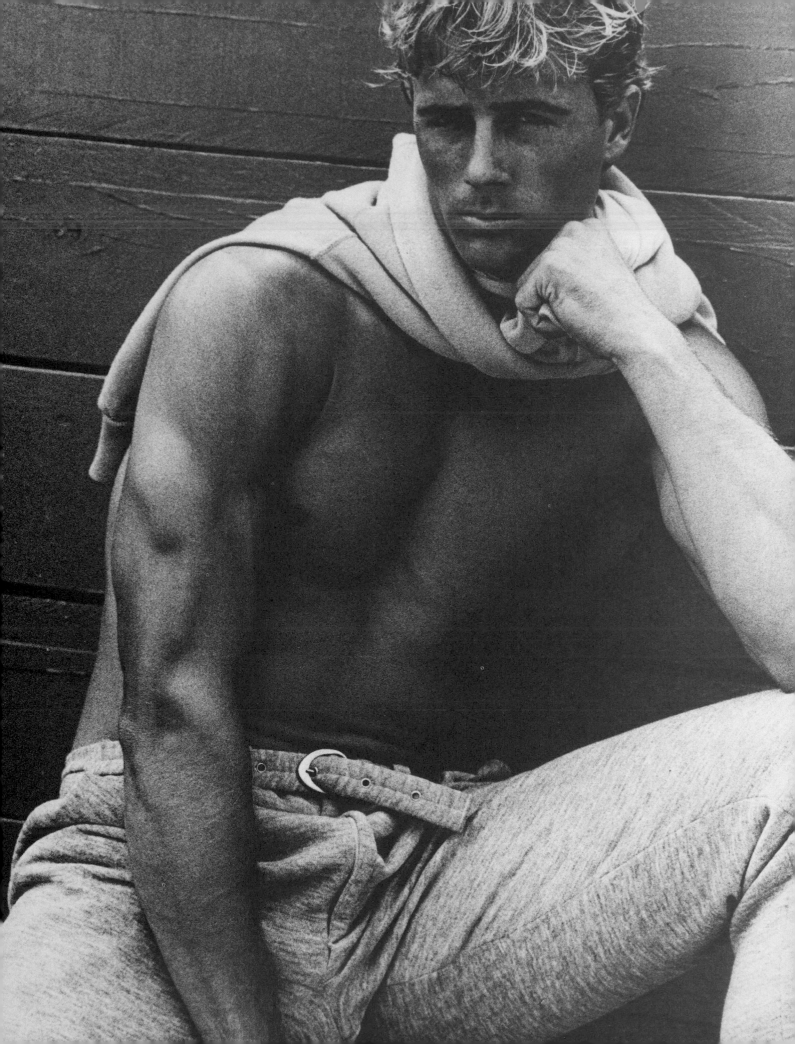

Your major decision concerns how many pounds you will allow your body to carry. The more you weigh, the more emphasis you must put on weight training. That emphasis, though, will become more intensive at later levels. During The Rookie Stage, just keep plugging away.

THE SINEWY BODY

Since your parents were genetically kind to you, you can build your body almost any way you want. The path of little resistance is to warm up and limber with gusto, then to improve your cardiovascular health to the hilt through aerobics. But since you've inherited the ability to add muscle more easily than most males, will you really be content to leave your physique relatively undeveloped?

First on the agenda is maintenance work to prime your body. Of the specific routines described in Chapter 6, Tracking (page 99) is especially effective for your body type.

Once you're rolling along at this exercise level, you must decide the degree of musculature you want to add to your frame. Merely to achieve a slender, lithe body, you won't need to lift any weights. Given your natural inclination to muscularity, calisthenics will give you good muscle definition. So

will light weights. But to achieve striking definition, the most efficient way is to concentrate on lifting heavier weights systematically from the beginning.

Another decision—albeit one to be made later down the exercise road—must be made regarding whether you aspire to specialized results. For example, if you want reasonably massive arms, you will put more emphasis on arm-building exercises. However, beware. Some men work out "what shows" (mainly arms and chest), ignoring "what's hidden" (their legs, for instance); they end up with physiques that look "mismatched" in their musculature. Given your innate advantage in body type, it's generally preferable to follow a well-rounded program, giving equal emphasis to all forms of exercise and to all parts of the physique.

THE STRINGY BODY

Building muscle mass is not the easiest for you, so if you want it, you're going to have to labor to get it. That way, against your natural inclination, you will eventually fill out your physique. But don't expect overnight results.

At this exercise level, your best bet is simply to follow all the routines religiously without making

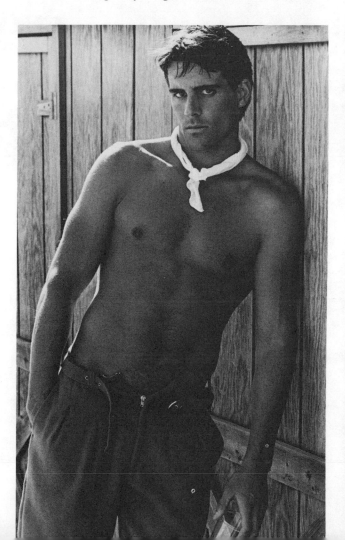

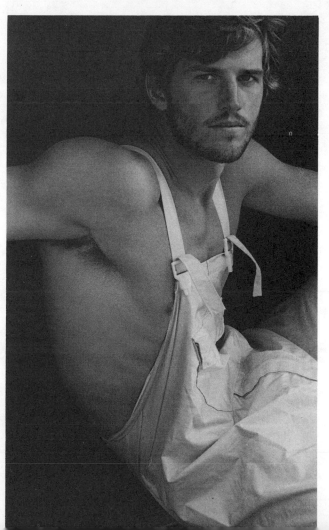

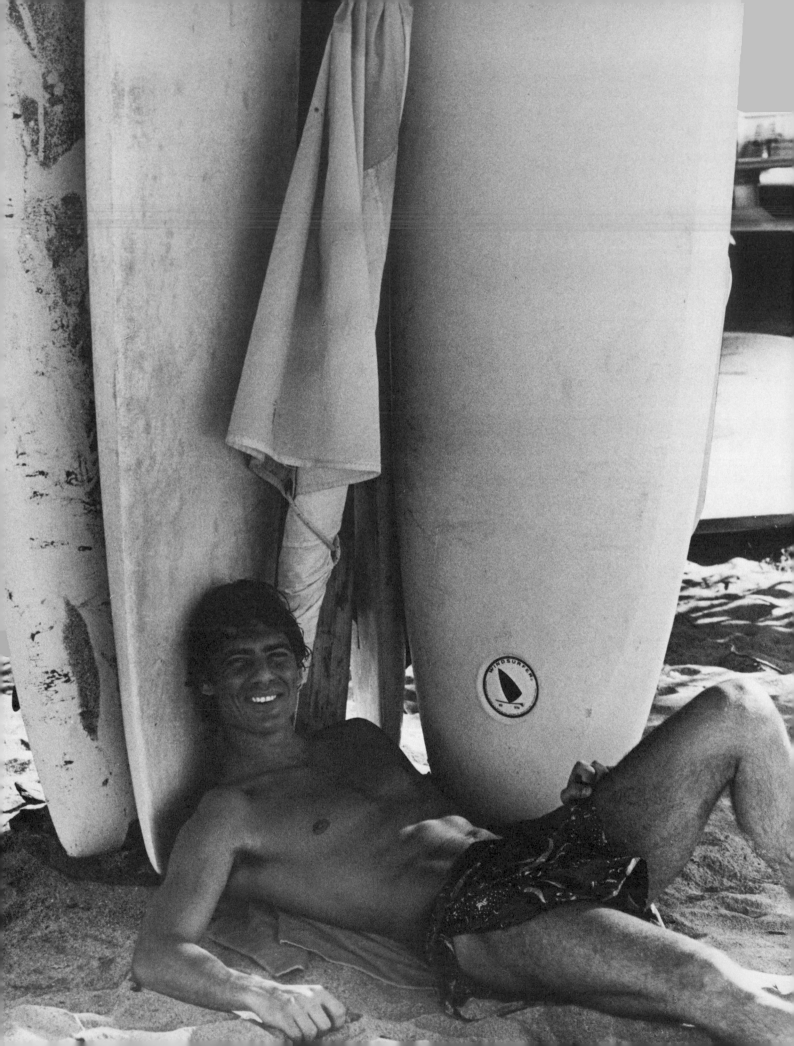

any major modifications. By sticking mainly to limbering exercises and doing the requisite aerobics, you will begin the gradual transformation of your contours. However, you should be careful with your maintenance exercises, because you don't want to lose weight. The less arduous, more fun ones—say, Twisting (page 96)—or the more literally calisthenics-inspired types—Swinging (page 97), for example—are best. Cycling is another good aerobic, particularly if you do it for long mileage at a less-than-furious pace. That way you won't burn off calories—and pounds—you may want to hold on to.

To make any dramatic changes in your physique, building exercises are a must. To begin with, simply do them all. Later, should you choose to emphasize certain parts of your body (your legs, for instance), increase the number of reps or sets specified. Meanwhile, stay committed, recognizing that weight training is your closest ally.

THE PLAYER STAGE

If you can start out at this stage in all categories of exercise, swell. That proves you're in "average" shape—which really means you're in better condition than most American males but you haven't achieved overall physical excellence yet. Why be content making an "average" impression if with some extra effort you can make a great one? Leap over the hurdle of your inertia and cover new ground.

But first take a few minutes to read the advice for fellows at The Rookie Stage. Do a few trial runs through those programs at the midway point. Are they truly easy for you? If you experience any difficulty, test your reactions to the routines earlier on. On the other hand, if they really are a snap, see how well you do at the end of all the programs in The Rookie Stage. If you can do them well with only a little or no difficulty, that's good, because the concluding level for The Rookie Stage is the entrance level for The Player Stage.

Of course, it may be that you're fine at the aerobics, not so fine at stretching, and just plain inexperienced with lifting weights. If so—or if you respond inconsistently in any other way—split your stages for the limbering, maintenance, and building routines.

TUNING EXERCISES

At this juncture, your cardiovascular fitness should be sufficient so you'll have to check your

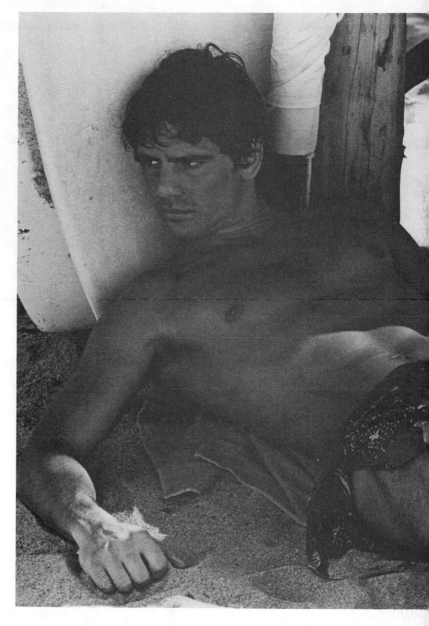

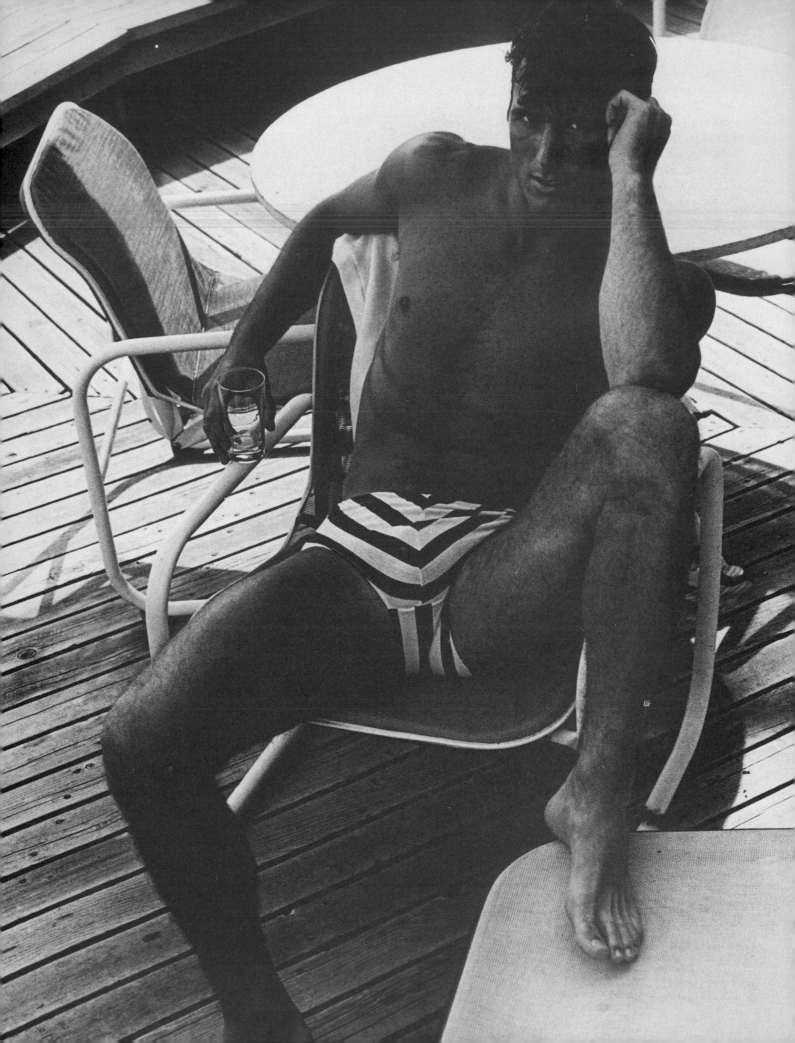

pulse only once, when you've nearly completed all sets of exercises, to make certain it's well below your training heartbeat.

All the warm-ups are now based on one set of five reps each, with approximately one minute (give or take a few seconds) allotted to each exercise set. Instead of opting for speed—which you should never do while tuning up—strive to perfect your form and improve your extension.

LIMBERING EXERCISES

Assuming you can execute the requisite five reps of all stretching exercises in a semblance of good form within fifteen minutes, tack on three more minutes of stretching for *a total of eighteen minutes of limbering.* Don't increase the number of reps; take a longer time doing every one of them, tensing and relaxing your muscles as you hold a stretch. Doing so really helps tone them.

And that's all you have to do while limbering during The Player Stage . . . other than constantly trying to improve your form, your coordination, and your agility while stretching and s-t-r-e-t-c-h-i-n-g smoother and s-m-o-o-t-h-e-r, breathing deeper and d-e-e-p-e-r.

MAINTENANCE EXERCISES

It isn't smart to pretend you're at The Player Stage if your cardiovascular system belies the fact. Aerobic fitness isn't something you toy with; you've got it or you ain't—with no room for bluff.

If you've reached the concluding level specified for The Rookie Stage—fifteen minutes of nonstop aerobic exercise without a heaving chest when finished—you're in pretty good shape. Now's the time for all good exercisers to come to their own aid and work out harder.

Maintaining a brisk but not brutal pace, *increase your maintenance session by three minutes to an eighteen-minute workout.* Do any combination of aerobics you choose as long as you move immediately from one to the next. Search for a perfect balance: Neither exceed your training heartbeat nor allow it to drop a beat lower. This means you'll have to measure it fairly often. Whenever your pulse begins to rise too high, slack off a little. If it then slows too much, give an extra push.

After eighteen minutes of aerobic work, cool down and call it a day.

After a few weeks at the eighteen-minute level, up your sessions to twenty minutes. Rely more strongly on your intuition to monitor your pulse. Still, to stay on the safe side, actually read it once or twice during the workout until you're positive your internal barometer is finely tuned.

With the passage of a couple more weeks, *start doing twenty-three-minute maintenance sessions.*

A month or two later, *ease up to twenty-five-minute periods.*

By now, your cardiovascular system should be showing marked improvement. And so should your body. To prove it to yourself, strip down to your briefs or nothing at all and spend a few minutes running in place before a full-length mirror. Admire the way your chest rises and descends rhythmically, the way your physique is toned. If you need any additional encouragement, dig out that photo of you taken before you started working out.

BUILDING EXERCISES

The fundamental changes in your building phase at this level will be technical: You continue doing the same exercises but with a new intensity.

Refer back to the chart on page 153. You'll note that by the conclusion of The Rookie Stage, the Intensity Routines specified require one set of ten reps for all the building exercises, with rest periods between the sets.

These are the modifications of the Intensity Routines to be followed during The Player Stage:

• Perform all the exercises as listed on the chart for *two sets of eight reps* each, resting briefly between each set and the next.

• Gradually eliminate the rest periods between the two sets of the same exercises. This is called *supersetting.*

• After a few weeks, perform all the exercises in *one set of ten reps each* and with *no* rest periods between *any* of the sets. This is called a *continuous circuit.*

Be advised, on your first forays using these new techniques, that you may not succeed in the nonstop fashion. You may have to use lighter weights than you've become accustomed to. Don't fret. Your body will adapt—no lie, it really will—and not too far down the road you'll not only be able to lift the same amount of weight again, you'll forge ahead by lifting even heavier weights than you are now doing. When this indeed occurs, increase your weights even more and really go to work. Do supersets during one session, the continuous circuit on others. Occasionally mix up your routines and put concentrated emphasis on various body parts on different days. If you don't vary your sessions, you

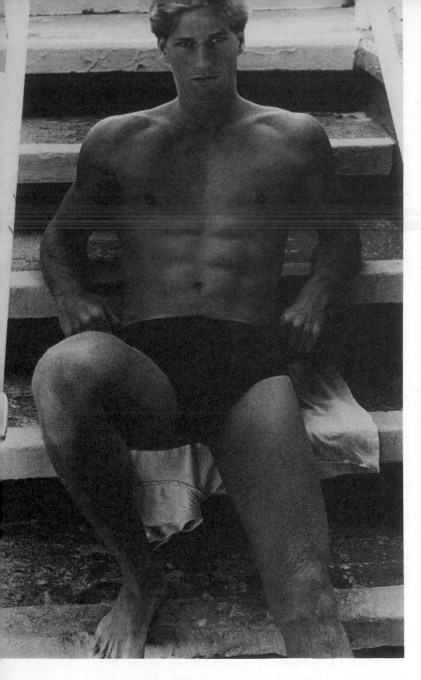

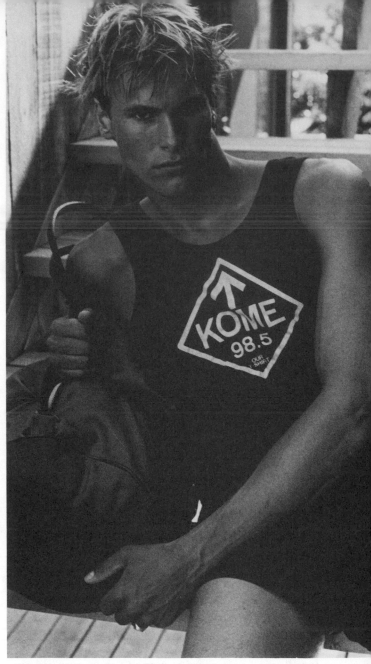

may find that you will plateau, that your muscles won't enlarge. In fact, that may happen anyway . . . but not for long if you keep challenging yourself in new ways. Getting into a rut is one way *not* to see the dimensional changes you desire.

Of course, once you've attained this level of performance, you've earned the right to do more than pat yourself on the back. Treat yourself to a long, steady look in the mirror. Bask in your accomplishments. Paste a solid-gold star on your forehead.

And step up to The Pro Stage.

COOLING EXERCISES

If you didn't perfect the cool-down movements at The Rookie Stage, do so now, always remembering they're to be done easily. If you need more than five-to-eight-minute sessions to regain your breath and normal heartbeat, that proves you've been really dedicated. Maybe too dedicated if you're drained.

When you have the exercises down pat, move directly to The Pro Stage. But earning a merit badge in cooling down is not worth cabling home about.

SUMMARY

When you're at The Player Stage of working out, your physical aspirations have more effect upon the modifications in your sessions. The following general program is only that—very general indeed. You will put your individual stamp upon it.

EVERY DAY

Tuning Exercises

You will now devote ten minutes to tuning up. This amount of time will remain consistent even as you step up the pace or length of your other phases.

Limbering Exercises

Increase your limbering sessions gradually over four weeks up to eighteen minutes.

Cooling Exercises

Allow seven or eight minutes for cooling down.

EVERY OTHER DAY

Maintenance Exercises

For the first two to four weeks at The Player Stage, advance to eighteen minutes of sustained aerobics.

Over the next two to four weeks, gradually increase your aerobic activity to twenty-minute sessions.

For the following month or two, raise the duration to twenty-five minutes.

Resistance Exercises

Unless you've decided to forgo them completely, devote thirty minutes throughout The Player Stage every other day to building exercises if you're intent upon developing strong musculature. (You can stretch out your building sessions longer if you feel comfortable doing so. Trust your body to tell you what's right for you, provided you don't overdo.)

So much for the general program at The Player Stage. Your daily workout time has increased very slightly to a steady sixty minutes a day. Now on to see what you'll do with that time considering your body type and your aims.

THE BURLY BODY

Once you've reached this exercise level, your particular physical aspirations come more into play. Fundamentally, the issue is the ratio between body fat and musculature.

If you've decided to battle your inbred inclination toward soft roundness and are intent upon keeping your weight down without seeking pronounced musculature, your workouts will not vary greatly from the rigors at the conclusion of The Rookie Stage. You will continue strong concentration on maintenance work to improve your cardiovascular fitness, and you will continue relatively lightly with building exercises primarily for body tone. You will not even graduate to The Player Stage in the building routines, and you will ignore supersets and the continuous circuit entirely. Lift weights only enough to keep—and not lose—your muscle definition. If you have an aversion to lifting weights, you can employ calisthenics to the same purpose.

On the other hand, if you've opted to tote around a few more pounds on your frame than the "average" athletic build might, you will require additional musculature to compensate for the extra girth. Otherwise you'll look paunchy. You must perfect all the building exercises and give more time to them if possible. At first, always allow a sufficient rest period between sets to regain your breath, but purposefully try to shorten these breathers as you progress. Attempt to work out more arduously every session by increasing your pace, doing more sets in a single time period. Here's how to modify the general program:

• Add five minutes of maintenance activity to that specified.
• Add five minutes of building activity.
• Subtract five minutes of limbering activity.

If you've set out to achieve specialized results, you may need to modify the general program further. Say you're on a quest for a massively muscled body to heave about in wrestlerlike dimensions. To transport that much body fat and still look attractive, you must court an equilibrium between your weight and your musculature, which means you'll require *big* muscles to accompany your large frame. And that means you'll have to work all that much harder. Toward the conclusion of The Player Stage, incorporate into your routine some of the techniques from The Pro Stage. Logically, for this type of look, you'll emphasize arm and chest muscles, so try doing two, even three sets of arm and chest exercises without a rest break. Or, if you're doing three sets of the same exercise, perform the second and third sets with heavier weights than the first. Here's how to modify the general program to accomplish this extra labor:

• Add five minutes of maintenance activity to that specified.
• Add ten minutes of building activity.
• Subtract five minutes of limbering.

In essence, use your logic. Once you enter The Player Stage, you will know what all the exercises do because the visual proof will be reflected in the mirror. You may still have a way to go, but you will also have come far. At that point, for extra proof, pull out the notebook where you entered all your measurements before you started working out and record your current tally. Cheers.

THE SINEWY BODY

You may not yet be the superb specimen you envision for yourself, but if you haven't been cutting corners, you should see marked improvement in your physique by the time you reach this plateau. After all, you're graced with the inborn ability to add muscle fairly easily.

Where do you head from here? That depends upon the decisions you made when you began this grand venture. If you have plotted vivid alterations in your physique, you're at a crossroads for a detour in strategy. If you've set out only to tone your body and add some muscle definition, just stay on course and don't get sidetracked.

The decision to change workout direction or not revolves around the musculature you're after and where you want those muscles to cling. If your goal is for overall development with only moderate definition, you can advance through all the steps at The Player Stage for the tuning, limbering, and maintenance phases without even embarking on the new discipline of the building phase. Ignore supersets and the continuous circuit entirely. Lift weights only enough to keep—and not lose—your muscle definition. If you have an aversion to lifting weights, you can employ calisthenics to the same purpose.

On the other hand, if you're seeking overall development *plus* strong muscle definition, the most efficient way to achieve this is by traveling step by step through the building phase as specified for this level.

Then again, should you be aiming for overall development and *chiseled* muscle definition, or for specifically bulging body parts, then you should start planning modifications in the general program. Initially, the most effective way for you to work out is by mastering the rigors of supersets and the continuous circuit. That will encourage fast development of your entire musculature. After that, once you're tooling along, you'll be able to tailor the sessions even more closely to your goals. Since your strength and endurance should both be much higher now, if you're specializing on leg and arm exercises, for example, get a jump on some of the techniques you'll encounter at The Pro Stage. Instead of doing one set of these exercises, do two without pausing

for a break. Also consider doing a second set with heavier weights than you used for the first. Or devote one entire session to nothing but leg and arm exercises. Here's how to modify the general program to accommodate this extra labor:

• Add ten minutes to your building activity.

In essence, use your logic. Once you enter The Player Stage, you will know what all the exercises do because the visual proof will be reflected in the mirror. You may still have a way to go, but you will also have come far. At that point, for extra proof, pull out the notebook where you entered all your measurements before you started working out and record your current tally. Cheers.

THE STRINGY BODY

If you can't see a major change in your body yet, don't be discouraged. Remind yourself that it's plain hard to build muscle on your body type. If you're not working *hard,* don't expect a transformation. If your physique is improving by leaps and bounds, hats off to you.

Your workout strategy during The Player Stage will be the same as in The Rookie Stage—more hard work, possibly with a few new refinements.

The decision to change workout direction or not revolves around the musculature you're after and where you want those muscles to cling. If your goal is overall development with only moderate definition, it's possible you may be in a position to advance through all the steps at The Player Stage for the tuning, limbering, and maintenance phases without even embarking on the new discipline of the building phase. That depends upon whether or not you achieved your desired muscle definition during The Rookie Stage. If your goal is for a slender, lithe body without emphatic musculature, that's occasionally possible to achieve via The Rookie Stage's building exercises. If you're fortunate, that will happen to you; you can then ignore supersets and the continuous circuit entirely if you choose. Lift weights only enough to keep—and not lose—your muscle definition. If you have an aversion to lifting weights, you can employ calisthenics to the same purpose.

If you do not achieve your desired muscle definition during The Rookie Stage, you must proceed step by step through the building phase as specified for this exercise level.

Weight training can also help with another difficulty. Given your body type, sometimes it's not only hard to increase muscles, it's also no easy trick to add meat to your bones. If your stringiness is

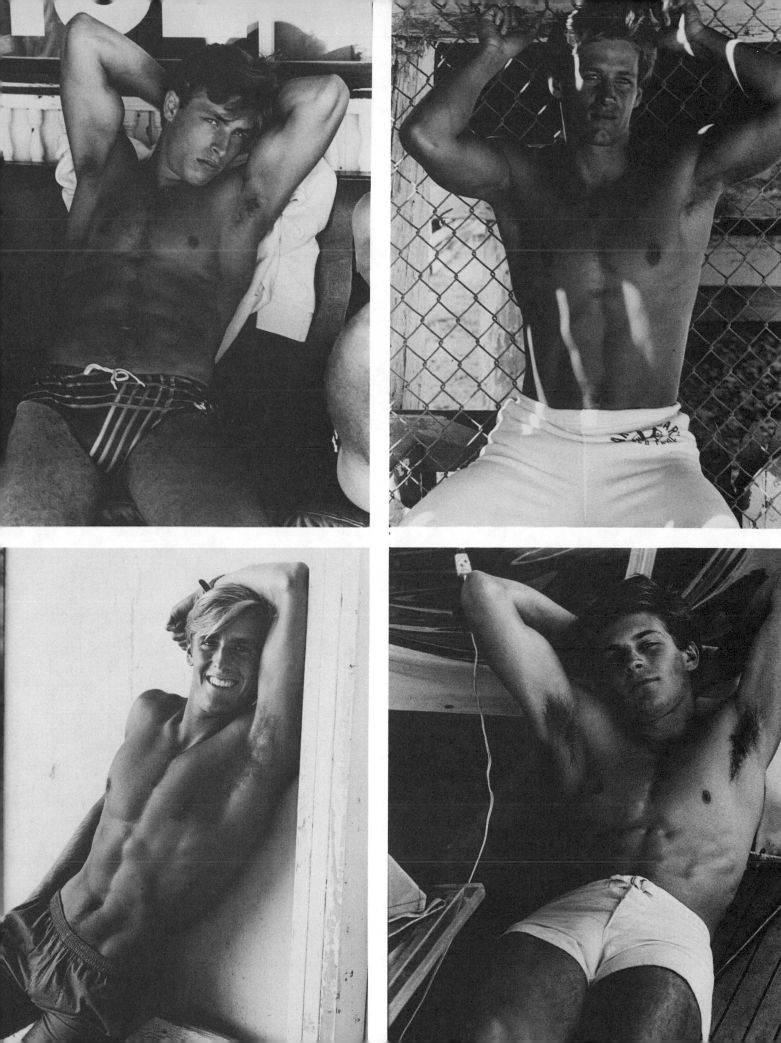

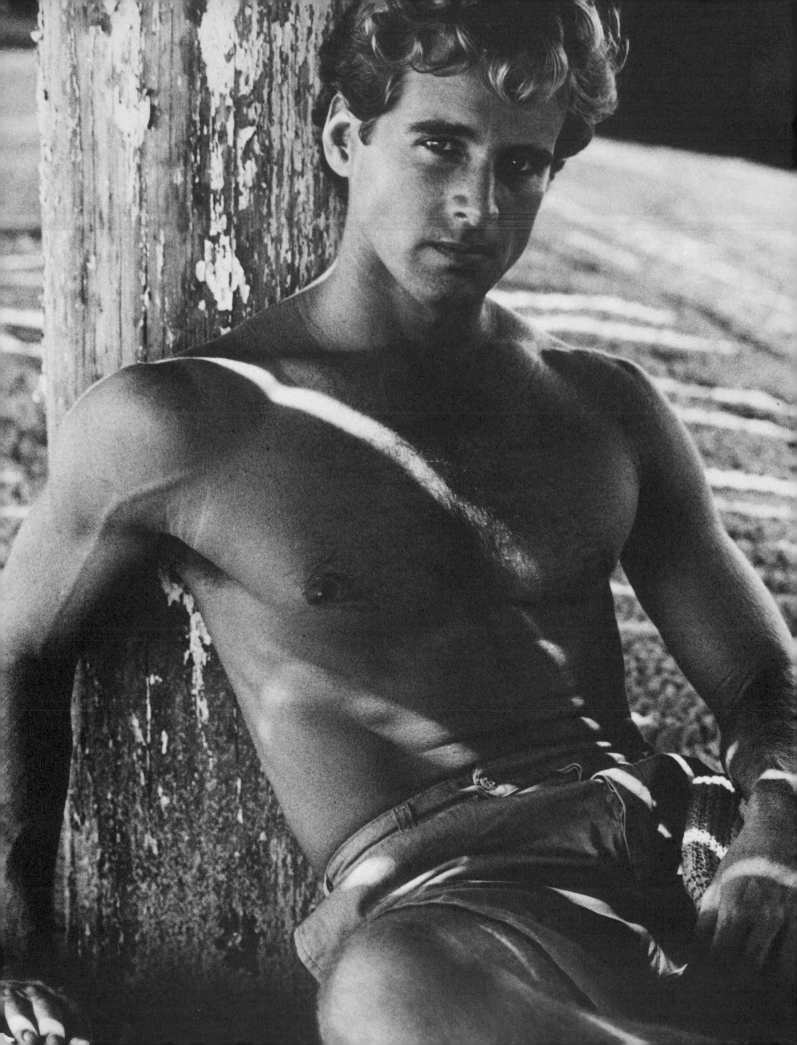

persisting, it could be that the austerity of your limbering and maintenance routines is preventing you from gaining the weight you may need to fill out your frame. One solution could be incorporating more building exercises.

Yes, lifting weights can help you gain weight if you plan it that way. Here's how.

Although most people gain weight in fat, if you purposefully increase your intake of healthful—not junk—food while also making a concerted effort to work out your major muscle groups, the weight you put on is mainly muscle. Oh, sure, some of it will also be fat, but when you cut back to your normal eating patterns, you'll probably lose about half the weight you gained—in the form of fat. So by eating more and exercising major muscles harder, you should contour your body.

Similarly, if you desire fairly defined musculature, you will also rely even more heavily on the new rituals of the building phase at this level as prescribed.

On the other hand, should you be aiming for overall development and *chiseled* muscle definition, or for specifically bulging body parts, then you should start planning modifications in the general program. Initially, the most effective way for you to work out is by mastering the rigors of supersets and the continuous circuit. That will encourage the most efficient development of your entire musculature. After that, once you're tooling along, you'll be able to tailor the sessions even more closely to your goals. Since your strength and endurance should both be much higher now, if you're specializing on leg and arm exercises, for example, get a jump on some of the techniques you'll encounter at The Pro Stage. Instead of doing one set of these exercises, do two without pausing for a break. Also consider doing a second set with heavier weights than you used for the first. Or devote one entire session to nothing but leg and arm exercises. Here's how to modify the general program to accommodate this extra labor:

• Subtract five minutes of limbering activity.
• Add ten minutes to your building activity.

In essence, use your logic. Once you enter The Player Stage, you will know what all the exercises do because the visual proof will be reflected in the mirror. You may still have a way to go, but you will also have come far. At that point, for extra proof, pull out the notebook where you entered all your measurements before you started working out and record your current tally. Cheers.

By the time you're nearing the end of The Player Stage, you should be a master at improvising your workouts.

THE PRO STAGE

Even if you've struggled to cross the border into this esteemed level, isn't your exhilaration at the vista worth the price of the passport?

TUNING EXERCISES

What more need you do with your warm-ups? Nothing. Just be certain you always do them and that you do them with the finest form you can muster. Never get sloppy or halfhearted when warming up. Always start off on the right foot with the right mental attitude. But you're a Pro, you know that. End of pep talk. Now go out there and dazzle the spectators.

LIMBERING EXERCISES

You must possess a high degree of agility to soar in at this level.

At The Player Stage, you peaked by doing all the limbering exercises in sets of five reps for a total of eighteen minutes. Since you're not racing against time, there's really no reason to do more than that —as long as you don't do less. On the other hand, if you enjoy stretching, tack on two more minutes to round off the session at *twenty minutes*. Extend your muscles even more fully during every exercise, tensing and relaxing them.

There's no reason to increase your reps, only your concentration. You might get bored repeating these same stretches? Easily remedied: Add some new ones of your own making. By now you can *feel* your individual muscles. Improvise whatever stretches appeal to you, on the proviso your entire body gets a workout.

By the way, how does it feel to be walking around with those fluid muscles of yours? Is that why you're smiling?

MAINTENANCE EXERCISES

As a Player you could do twenty-five minutes of maintenance exercises comfortably. Now that you're a Pro, the big time is *thirty minutes* of go-gogoing aerobic work at your training heartbeat every other day. Now and again, you may opt to speed up even faster for a few minutes just to prove you can. No harm done if your pulse stays below your maximum safe heart rate. The payoff of shaping up is a body worth showing off.

If you've become an aerobics addict in the process, fine. Work out to your heart's and emotions' content. As long as you're aware of your training heartbeat, you just can't overindulge. All you'll do is get better. And better. Year after year.

BUILDING EXERCISES

From here on, your building exercises are a series of refinements. But if you're cutting in at The Pro Stage without going through the ranks, it's imperative that you have a high level of expertise. To be extra-certain, go back and read the building section of The Player Stage. The routines are not exactly fluff.

Stick with supersets and the continuous circuit for as long as you like, increasing weights if you choose. However, the amount of weight you can lift is finite. It's okay to push yourself, but not to the point of absurdity.

Consider other factors too. How muscular do you truly want to be? If you want brim atop brim of muscles, just pump away. Do you want to improve some parts of your body more than others? If so, start specializing. Have you already reached the body proportions you desire? In that happy circumstance, just keep doing what you're already doing without laboring any harder.

Depending upon your goals, your options are many. Because you have to be in excellent shape to be inducted into The Pro Stage, you no longer have to work out your entire body every building session, as long as you're conscientious and don't permit any body area to backslide. Figuratively cutting your body in half and alternating two types of workouts is the best way to get more specialized results. For one session, concentrate on the muscles on the top part of your body—your neck, shoulders, arms, chest, and upper back; for the other session, concentrate on the bottom half—your lower back, waist, abdomen, buttocks, and legs.

Split Body Routine

Perform all the exercises listed in the Intensity Routines chart on page 153 down to and including the Chest, plus The Row-Down and The Deadlift (both affecting the upper back), on Day 1.

On Day 2, starting with The Dumb Row and The Row-Down (both affecting the lower back), complete the exercises listed from the Waist through the Legs.

Although this sounds as if you're exercising your body areas only half often as previously, don't forget that the *intensity of labor* you put into every session affects the outcome. Also, when you realize that you will be doing more reps per exercise set than you've ever attempted to date, it becomes obvious you won't be letting up. In fact, by working out half your muscles much, much harder, you'll be pushing them to their limits of endurance, exhausting and enlarging them. By giving them a longer rest between sessions, you afford them more recovery time so you can work them that much harder when you zero in on them again. Never lose sight of the fact that there is only so much work your muscles can do, and if you're absolutely relentless with them without letting them heal from the workout traumas, they'll break down instead of building up.

In your split body routine, although you'll be varying the exercises, you can set the same goals for each session. Start out doing two sets each of ten reps, with brief stretching periods between the two sets and a longer rest between each group of exercises and the next for the different body parts.

After a few weeks, superset each set, eliminating the short stretches.

A few weeks later, consider all the exercises for each part of the body as a circuit. Perform them continuously. Naturally, you'll take time after each circuit to regain your breath and lower your pulse.

Now you can choose whether to increase your reps in each set or to increase the amount of weight you're using. Still later on, you might choose to do both.

If this plan isn't to your liking, adapt it. Maybe you'll make a partial split during your sessions, beginning each period with a total body workout, then zeroing in on particular parts of the body for two or three sets of ten reps. That way you'll be altering the ratio of your exercises by selectively increasing the number of reps and the intensity of certain exercises.

Partial Split Routines

On Day 1, with the primary focus on the upper body, perform the following exercises in the following order.

NECK: The Weighted Shrug—page 107
SHOULDERS: The Dip—page 111

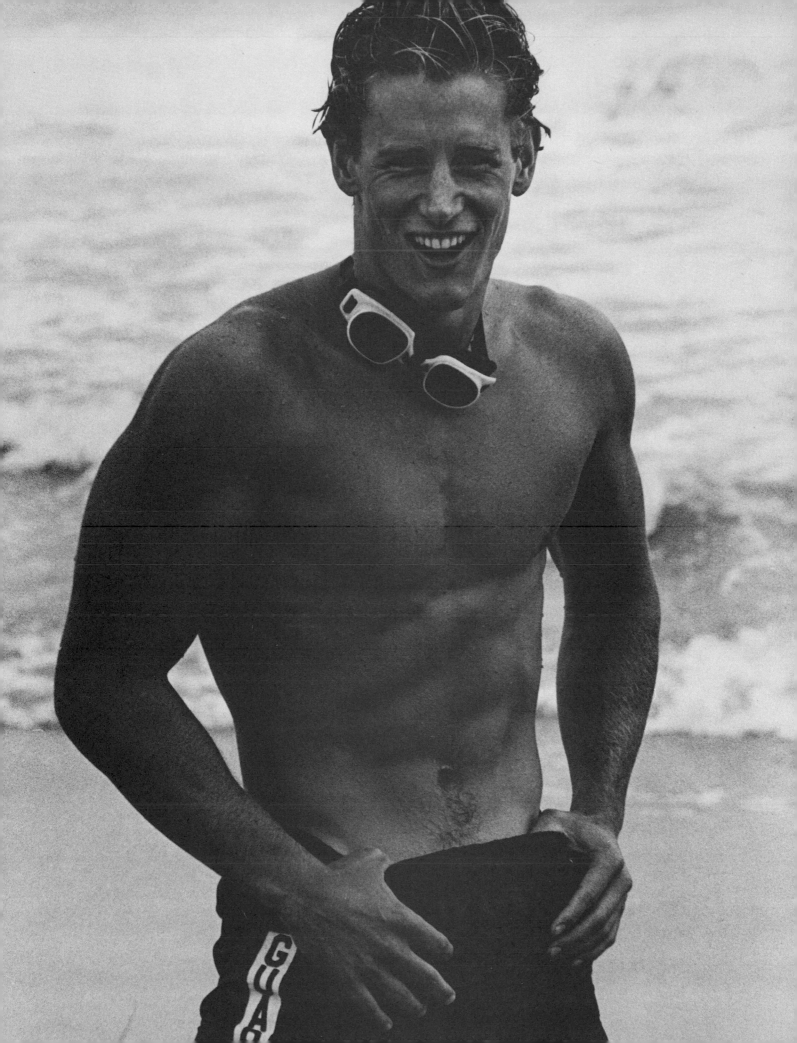

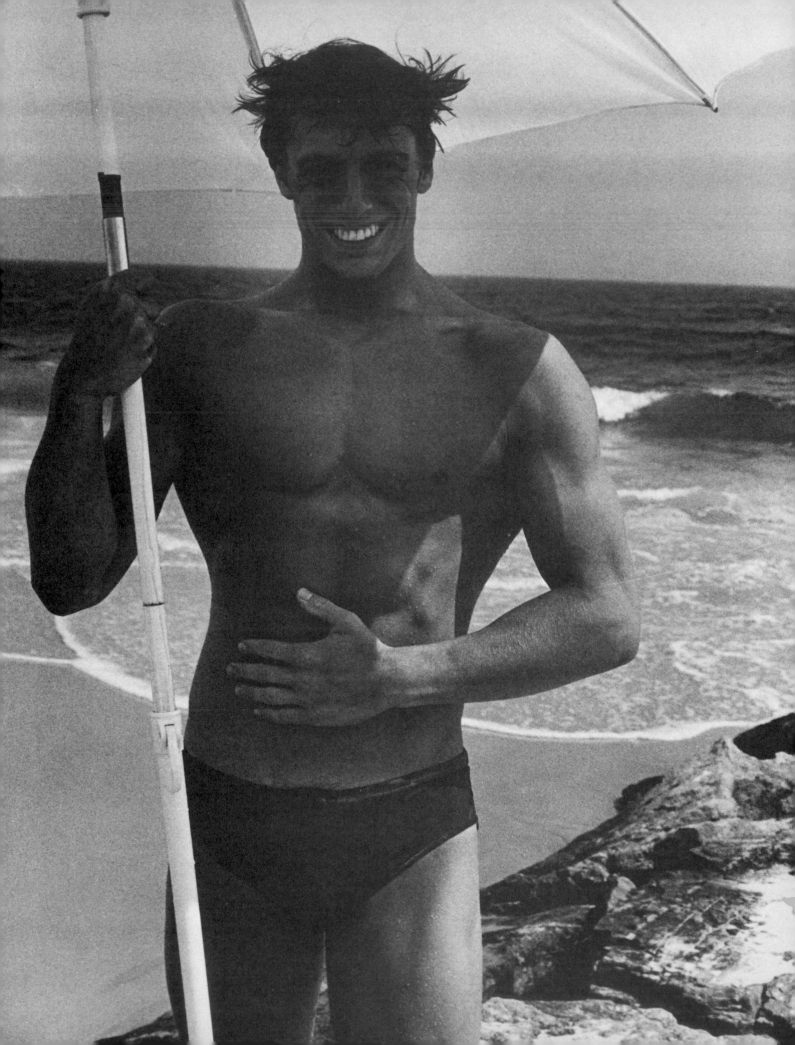

ARMS: The Curl I—page 115
The Extension I—page 118
CHEST: The Push-Off—page 121
LOWER BACK: The Dumb Row—page 125
WAIST: The Dumb Bend—page 129
ABDOMEN: The Ankle-Up—page 133
BUTTOCKS: The Swing—page 137
LEGS: The Toe-the-Line—page 141
The Lunge-Up—page 143
NECK: The Lift-and-Shrug—page 108
The Row-Up—page 109
SHOULDERS: The Press-Back—page 112
The Dumb Lat—page 113
ARMS: The Curl II—page 116
The Curl III—page 117
The Extension II—page 119
CHEST: The Dumb Fly—page 122
The Dumb Over—page 123
UPPER BACK: The Row-Down—page 126
The Deadlift—page 127

On Day 2, with primary focus on the lower body, perform the following exercises in the following order.

UPPER BACK: The Deadlift—page 127
WAIST: The Dumb Bend—page 129
ABDOMEN: The Ankle-Up—page 133
BUTTOCKS: The Swing—page 137
LEGS: The Toe-the-Line—page 141
NECK: The Weighted Shrug—page 107
ARMS: The Curl III—page 117
The Extension II—page 119
CHEST: The Push-Off—page 121
LOWER BACK: The Dumb Row—page 125
The Row-Down—page 126
WAIST The Seated Twist—page 130
The Bent Twist—page 131
ABDOMEN: The Knee-Up—page 134
The Back-Up—page 135
BUTTOCKS: The Kick—page 138
The Kneel—page 139
LEGS: The Up-Front Squat—page 142
The Lunge-Up—page 143

At this level you might also want to add more weights for each set within a circuit. This excellent ploy always keeps you moving ahead.

Or you might improvise an entirely different schedule.

In other words, at The Pro Stage, you've earned the right—and the discipline—to be responsible for yourself. And you've also earned a laurel wreath. Congratulations.

COOLING EXERCISES

When you've been going hot and heavy, sometimes it takes more than ten minutes to become cool and light. As a Pro, you'll be professional about getting yourself back under control.

SUMMARY

Once you've made it to The Pro Stage, you should be so aware of your body that instinct will tell you what improvisations to make. Merely to maintain your excellent physical status, continue the regimens you developed by the conclusion of The Player Stage. In pursuit of greater excellence, however, you will work out even harder. But considering your terrific condition, it won't seem as if you're expending all that much more labor.

You will vary the general program, adapting it to your own needs, but here it is as a starting point for The Pro Stage.

EVERY DAY

Tuning Exercises

Give yourself a good eight minutes.

Limbering Exercises

Twenty minutes is the minimum. Devoting more time is preferable.

Cooling Exercises

Take ten minutes.

EVERY OTHER DAY

Maintenance Exercises

Over a four-to-six-week period, work up to a minimum of thirty minutes of nonstop aerobic activity each session.

After attaining this level, you can endure any amount of aerobic exercise you like as long as you don't exceed your maximum safe heartbeat.

Building Exercises

Over two to four weeks, gradually increase your resistance phase to forty minutes.

Taking another two to four weeks, build up to fifty-minute sessions.

The following two to four weeks, work up to hourly sessions every other day.

After achieving this level, trust your body to inform you when you should call a halt to your resistance workout.

Of course, you will probably modify this general program to achieve your specific aims. Your daily regimen will now vary in length from a bit more than an hour to an hour and a half . . . if you want to go the most comprehensive route. If you can't afford the time, pare down some of the routines, always exerting maximal intensity. Try to compress as much disciplined labor as possible into each session. Don't forget, the harder you work out within a given time span, the greater the rewards.

THE BURLY BODY

The acronym of wisdom: MOS (More Of Same).

There's no new message for you that wasn't implicit in the wrap-up following The Player Stage. Simply review your resolutions and your results to date.

If your initial goal was simply to watch your weight and tone your muscles, you should already have accomplished it. If you haven't, you've been cheating—or overeating—somewhere along the line. Start over again at The Player Stage and stick to it!

If you still want specialized results—such as titanic thighs—use all the sophisticated techniques of The Pro Stage to get them.

THE SINEWY BODY

At this plateau you're expecting a whole set of new directions? Don't. And unless you've drastically rearranged your priorities, you don't need any.

As you're now in tip-top condition, one more strip before a full-length mirror should be the validation and your vindication.

If your body isn't all you want it to be, the most serious failing is probably in the building routines. Proceed back to that section of The Player Stage and begin again with gusto. But don't short-change yourself in the maintenance or limbering routines.

If you're after very specialized goals—a chest to end all chests, for instance—plow ahead with split body routines for the upper body.

THE STRINGY BODY

What more do you need to know? That's not a rhetorical question. Think about it.

After completing both The Rookie and The Player Stages, you reexamined your priorities. At this level of excellence, all the tools you need are at your disposal.

Take one more long, hard look at your body. If you've been conscientious, your body should look hard and long too. If it doesn't, don't give up. Add yet more variety to your workouts. One session, use a split body routine. Next session, go for the continuous circuit. You've got the ability and the means, so have fun. Keep sight of your goals and you'll attain them.

Once you've attained The Pro Stage, as a reminder of how far you've come, think back to when you began. Visualize your step-by-step improvement. You did it all by yourself. For yourself.

And that, in a very sizable nutshell, is all you need to know about working out unless you want to turn it into an obsession. Don't. Moderation is much more flattering than fanaticism.

Although smugness isn't a virtue, when you're working out at The Pro Stage, call up a friend who has a good camera and a photogenic eye. For posterity—and for all your distant friends and relatives who haven't seen you since you took the plunge—record in living color the *real* you who has materialized from your imagination. After sending that photo around, to atone for your hubris . . . Hell, don't repent. A *little* smugness never hurts. Then again, neither does a little humility. The way you'll look after entering The Pro Stage, your physique will speak for itself. Loud and clear.

SELF CENTERED

When you've worked out and shaped up, don't dilute the impact of your success by haphazard grooming. Even before you reach that blissful stage, you can make more of yourself through exacting personal care. Read on.

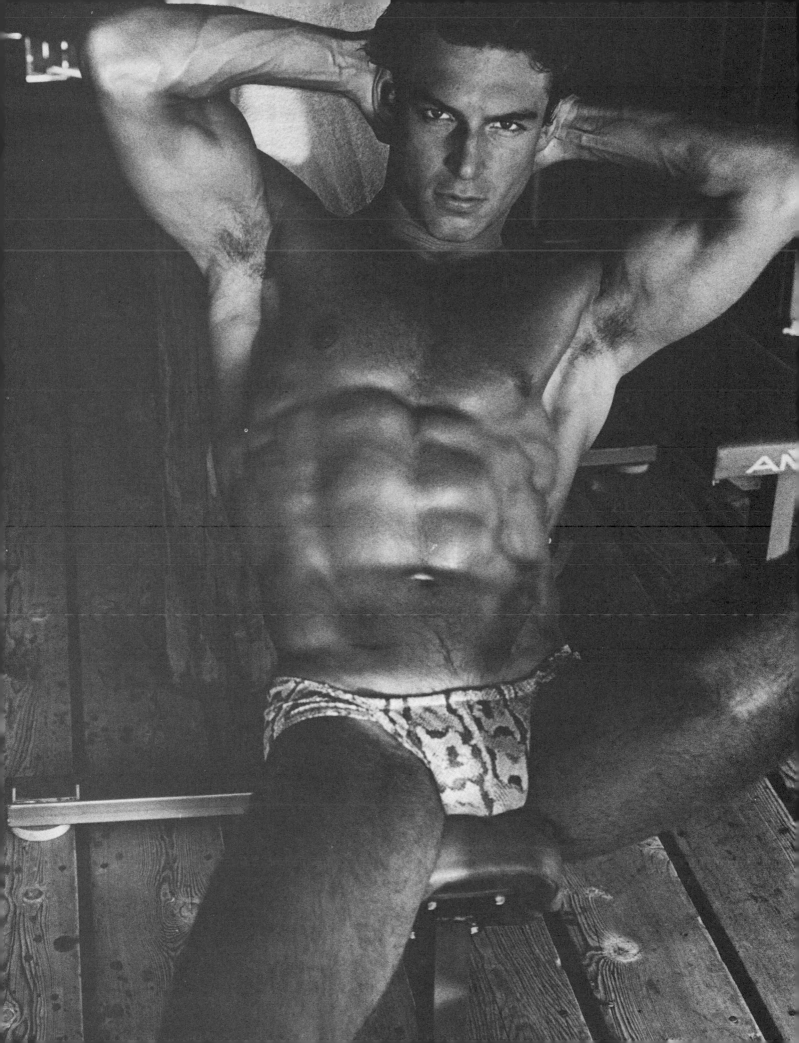

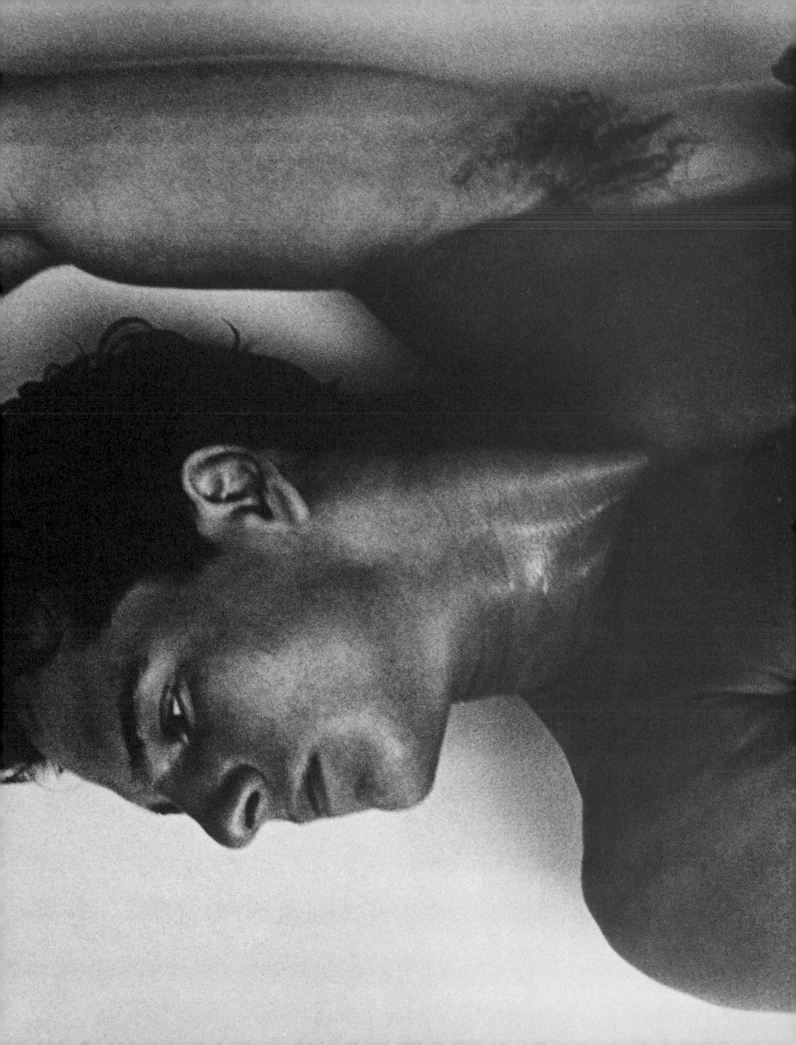

PART III

PRIDE &
GROOM

CHAPTER 9

MANE THING

IN A LATHER

Whenever you take a sweat bath, your hair is among the first to know. Perspiration being little more than salt water with some waste thrown in, it coats your hair with salt whenever you reach a dripping state. That salty solution immediately starts attacking your hair.

On the other hand, when you've worked yourself into a lather, your nervous system orders oil glands all over the body, including the scalp, to start pumping their reserves. These oils fend off the aggressive salt for a while. If you stop exercising at this strategic point, your hair will probably end up oilier than usual. However, the more you keep plugging away, the more likely that salt will be victorious. Your hair will be drier—less protected by natural oils—than normal at the end of your workout. To compensate for any detrimental effect, and to normalize your hair as much as possible, it's wise to shampoo after a vigorous exercise session.

But a slipshod shampoo is a shoddy remedy.

Shampooing accomplishes more than the removal of salt. It also eliminates pollutants and other accumulations from the environment . . . and strips away oils protecting the hair shaft. (Ironically, hair needs a bodyguard because it's dead. More about that ghoulish fact shortly.) If you have dry hair to begin with, whenever you wash your hair, it gets even drier. Conversely, if you have oily hair, shampooing can help neutralize that by removing oil excess.

To do your hair a favor, you must recognize its natural (pre-exercise) state. Is it oily? dry? or normal?

OILY HAIR. It gets dirty fast because invisible-to-the-eye airborne debris sticks to the oil; it quickly looks greasy when unshampooed.

DRY HAIR. Lacking a healthy amount of oil to give it luster and a natural sheen, it looks lifeless when left on its own.

NORMAL HAIR. It looks, not very surprisingly, normal. It isn't greasy and it isn't dull; it's healthy-looking.

To get a clearer fix on efficacious hair care, take a closer look at your hair. Peer so closely, in fact, that if you weren't imaginative, you would require a high-power microscope.

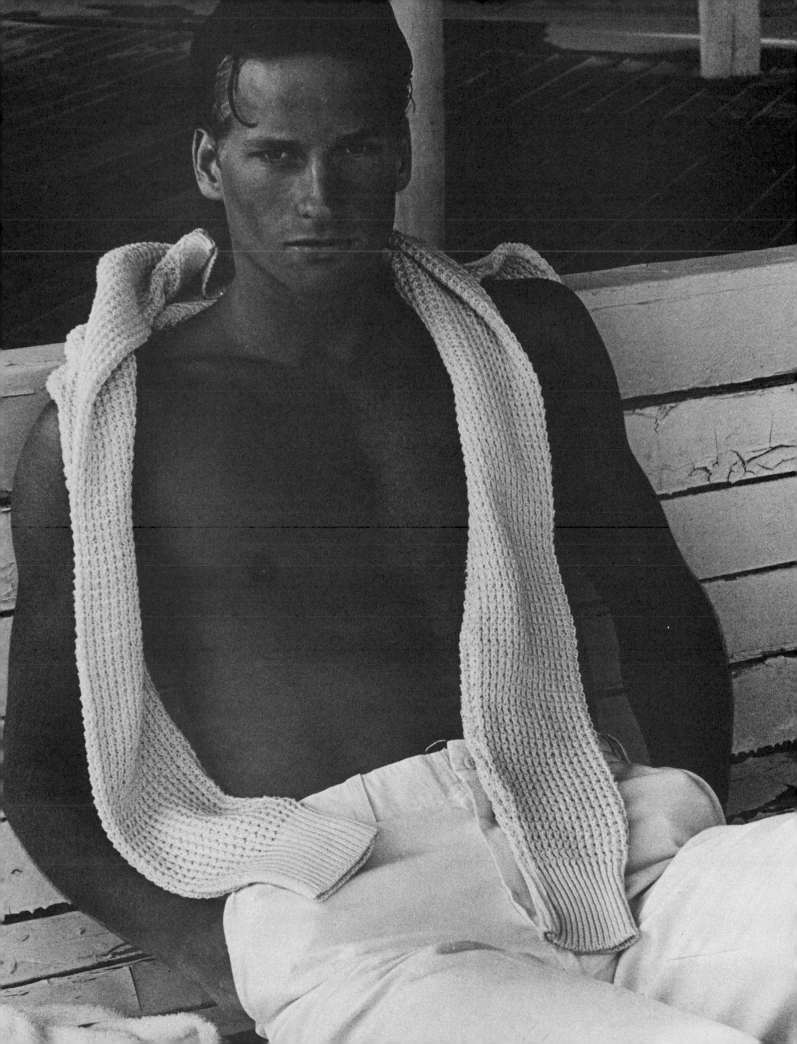

OVER VIEW

Now for the morbid truth about hair. All the individual strands (called *shafts*) are defunct—nothing more than unwanted waste material pushed from beneath the scalp's surface in an effort to be rid of it.

Every strand has a root that's small but active (provided it is among the living). Most of the root activity takes place in a tiny sac named the *follicle*. At the base of the follicle is an even smaller "bud" called the *papilla*. When people commonly refer to the hair root, they're really talking about the papilla, which grows hair throughout its lifetime.

Papillae are responsible for creating new protein cells within the follicles. As these new cells are formed, the older ones are pushed up through the pore openings of the scalp. While beneath the skin, these cells are nourished by blood, but once they are exposed, their source of nourishment is no longer handy. They expire, becoming part of the hair shaft.

Back below the surface, residing near every hair follicle, are oil-producing glands known as *sebaceous glands*. They produce the oil secretions that lubricate and protect the defunct hair shafts. (Actually, they also produce the oils found all over the surface of the body to protect the skin as well.) If these glands are hyperactive, the result is oily hair. If they're sluggish, dry hair ensues. When they're pumping normally, the hair is normal.

To the surface again. The hair shaft is usually composed of three layers: The *cuticle* (outer) layer, consisting of overlapping cells reminiscent of fish scales with empty spaces between them; the *cortex* (middle) layer which contains the color-imparting pigments, principally melanin; and the *medula* (core), which is essentially a hollow tube of unknown significance. Many hair shafts have no medulas and aren't at all upset by the lack.

Fading hair color signifies slower melanin production. White hair has no pigment. Different shafts contain differing amounts and combinations of pigment, so no head of hair is all one consistent shade.

Below-the-surface hair growth is fairly cyclical. Each scalp hair grows for an average of four years or so, then rests for about three months. When this resting phase is over, the papilla starts forming cells anew, pushing out the older hair shaft that had sprouted from the same root. That's why some daily hair loss—approximately fifty shafts a day—is actually a healthy sign, indicating ongoing hair replenishment. This shedding is hardly dramatic, since more than 100,000 hair follicles are found on the average head.

If follicles worked in unison—which they don't—you would molt, becoming totally bald about every four years. Three months or so later, you'd start growing hair again. As it is, however, many more follicles are always active than resting, with a "full" head of hair the visible consequence . . . as long as baldness doesn't complicate matters. As men age, regrowth slows down, accelerating recession.

Accumulations of male sex hormones in the bloodstream also affect hair growth, because when the level is high, hair goes into its resting stage whether or not the time is right. As the hormonal level continues to increase, so do the resting cycles. This inactivity causes the papillae to atrophy and eventually die.

Although male sex hormones do the papillae in, the real assassins are genes. Male pattern baldness is a genetic condition, and if you have inherited it, not one federally funded scientific study suggests there's anything you can do to get around it. But baldness isn't a dread disease; it's a fact of life for some men and not for others. And that's that.

HAIR APPARENT

Understanding hair's structure helps you separate fact from fiction. For instance, think about the tall tale that shampooing every day makes you lose your hair faster. That's pure fiction, because (a) unless you're washing your hair with sulfuric acid, no shampoo formula will bore through your scalp to attack the papillae, and (b) balding is the result of genetics, not shampooing.

Although it sounds radical, unless your scalp becomes so encased in grime that the metabolism of the papillae is affected, hair cleanliness is really only a cosmetic consideration. You don't shampoo to make your hair healthier or to keep it longer; you shampoo to look better. Touchable hair is attractive; filthy hair isn't. Hair sprayed to a lacquerlike finish is neither touchable nor attractive because it doesn't feel or look natural.

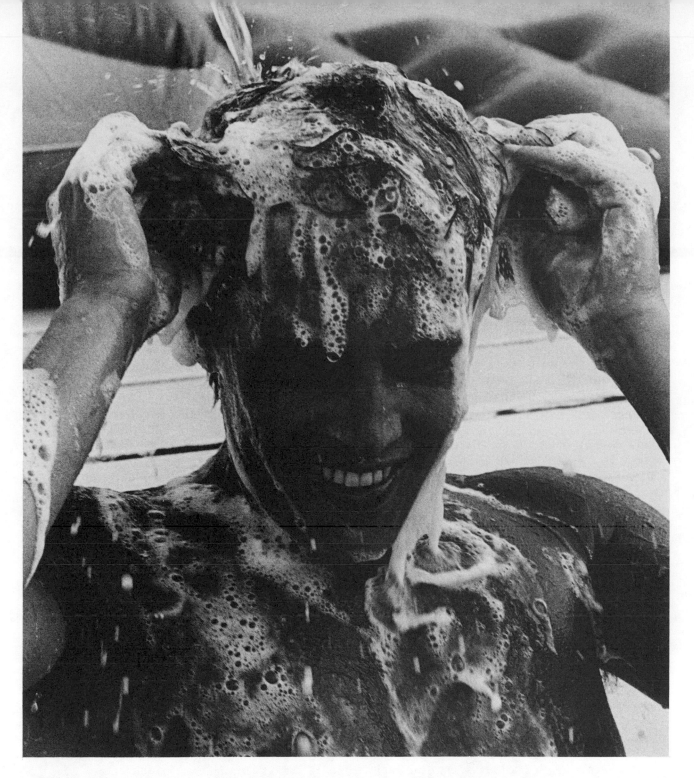

For hair to look and feel natural, you can't ignore it after your workout. Here are a few points to keep in mind.

SHAMPOOING

Once you undertake a shape-up program, you're committing yourself to a daily shampoo because of all the sweat, literal and metaphoric, involved. De-

pending upon when you work out and the condition of your hair, you may decide to shampoo twice a day.

Before tackling that logistical problem, let's first clear up the question of what shampoo to use.

Need you purchase one with exotic ingredients and an astounding price tag? No. Your sole interest is aesthetic results. Any shampoo that leaves your hair looking good is the right one for you. Experiment. Look in the mirror. If your hair looks swell after shampooing with an inexpensive brand, why pay more? You can't mortally injure hair that's already dead. But you can enhance its appearance or detract from it. Keep those eyes open.

If you have dry hair, you will probably choose the gentlest shampoo you can locate; products formulated for the dry condition are among the gentlest.

With normal hair and a once-a-day shampoo schedule, a product formulated for normal (or average) hair will likely be your best bet. However, when shampooing twice a day, try a product formulated for dry hair. You could strip away too much oil with a more concentrated formula on a twice-a-day shampooing frequency.

Oily hair and a once-a-day shampoo regimen? Presumably you'll require the strength of a product formulated for that condition. If your hair is exceedingly oily, you still might use the same oily-hair concentration when shampooing it twice daily. But if your hair is only slightly oily, consider using a shampoo formulated for normal hair in a twice-a-day routine.

How do you determine how often to shampoo? By how you want your hair to look, and by when you want it to look that way. And that depends upon the individual way your hair reacts. Some guys wake up in the morning with their hair impersonating a rat's nest. Only shampooing will tame their wayward mane. For others, a quick rinse with water, a fast dry with a towel, and a rapid flick of a comb will make their hair look as if they'd just stepped out of a tonsorial parlor. Some guys are even luckier; they can stumble out of bed, arrange their hair with their fingertips, and look presentable

to royalty. How your hair reacts throughout the day —but especially at wake-up time—offers the care clues.

If you exercise before heading for work, the simplest routine is shampooing after the workout. (Handsomely styled and squeaky-clean hair isn't mandated before working out. Hard work will soon undo styling and cleanliness efforts.) You probably won't need to shampoo again that entire day because you probably won't work yourself into a sweat again. However, if you do or if for any reason your hair gets very dirty, then you'll shampoo a second time before stepping out on the town.

Exercising at midday makes it more difficult to calculate when to wash your hair. Unless you're the lucky kind of fellow who can sleep, arise, put a comb through his hair, and still look well groomed. In that fortunate event, you could get by with only one daily shampoo, following the midday workout.

If you have very oily hair, the drying effects of the salt on the hair aren't all that terrible. If you rinse your hair thoroughly with lots of water—and if your hair still looks good with this minimal ministration—then don't shampoo after the midday workout. When should you wash your hair? Whenever you choose, as long as it looks good when you want it to.

With dry or normal hair, you should allocate the extra time to shampoo after the midday session, because even an extra-long water rinse might not whirl away all the drying salt. You must be extra-cautious. At other times, if your hair needs additional attention that a water rinse will satisfy, don't subject it to another shampoo. *Unless* . . . (A couple of new strategies are coming up in a few seconds.)

HAIR REPLACEMENT

Even before Delilah clipped Samson, charlatans were hawking miraculous hair restorers. Their disreputable descendants are still offering empty promises at fully inflated prices. Once the hair root kicks the bucket, hair revitalization is a dead issue.

Men who psychologically can't adjust to baldness should look for help not from con men but from companies selling hairpieces. *But*—and here's the big reservation—hair replacements and exercising don't mix.

Whenever a man exercises while wearing a hairpiece, scalp perspiration is trapped beneath the piece. Evaporation is hindered. Bacteria grow. The potential for scalp irritation grows too.

Even on an aesthetic level, hair replacements don't team up with working out. Because of all the scalp perspiration, whatever hair of his own a man has left becomes drenched and responds to the wetness in its own way. The replacement hair may or may not get wet, and responds in *its* own way, differently from the fringe of authentic hair, making it perfectly obvious that the fellow is wearing a rug. There's no such thing as a good cover-up if someone can detect it.

If you wear a hairpiece, always remove it before working out. You might even think about tossing out the piece permanently. So what if recession makes you look a little older? Once your physique is shaped up, maturity and muscularity can be irresistible.

What if you exercise after work? If your hair looks fine without shampooing *before* work, then shampooing after the workout will suffice. If your hair just doesn't look its best unless you shampoo it after rolling out of bed, then shampoo after rising *and* after exercising, even with dry hair.

To repeat, how your hair looks is the ultimate criterion. And how it looks isn't solely dependent upon shampooing. Even when you're conscientious, shampooing can take its toll. Your hair can lose its luster. Or stubbornly resist your comb.

Welcome to the world of hair conditioners. Shampooing is only the first step in hair care, and what you do in the second or third can affect the initial one.

CONDITIONING

Remember the way the outer layer of the hair shaft is made up of fishlike scales? Well, that fact affects hair appearance before and after shampooing.

Between those scales are air pockets. Hair oils help hold the scales together, reducing the volume of the open spaces. When hair oil is whisked away by a thorough shampooing, hair can look flyaway because the scales may open too wide. In turn, that can cause hair shafts to tangle, as the scales of one shaft catch the scales of another.

So-called hair conditioners are designed to seal the fishlike scales on the hair shaft to restore natural shine and make the hair more manageable. Some also reduce static and restore softness. Generally applied after shampooing, most conditioners are of an oily or creamy consistency. They are usually worked into the wet (or partially wet) hair, then rinsed away with water, leaving deposits only between the scales on the hair shaft.

Here's the paradox about shampooing and conditioning. When your hair starts reacting negatively

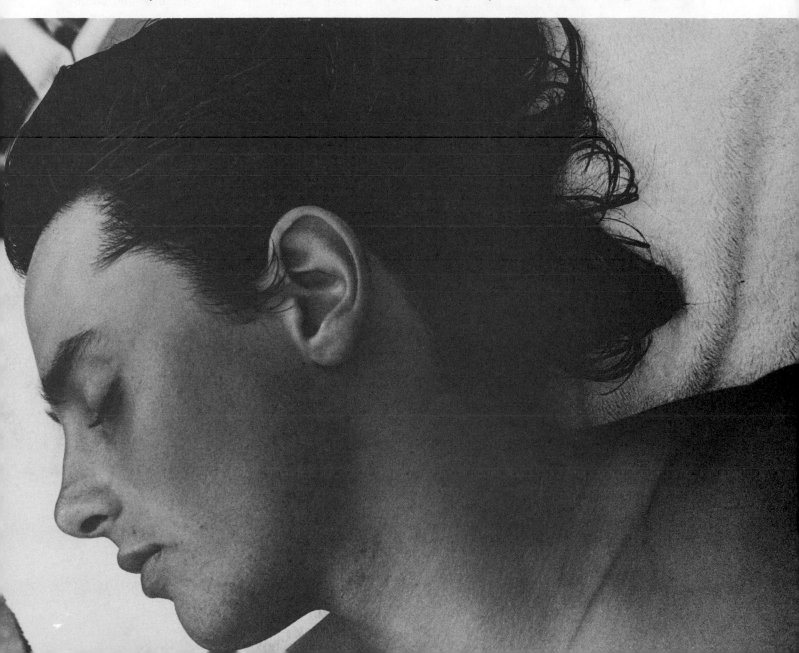

to a shampoo, you'd think it smarter to lather up less often, right? Only partially right. If no corrective measure is taken, you *do* risk shampooing too often. But if you apply a conditioner afterward, shampooing more often is no problem. So even with very dry hair, you can still shampoo twice a day *if* you also condition your hair twice a day.

With normal hair, you need condition your hair only occasionally when using a shampoo with the correct formulation.

GOING GRAY

Like a receding hairline, going gray never proclaims the decline and fall of man, unless you're the man going gray and you're not ready to accept it. Nobody's stopping you from having your gray retouched. But if you do resort to artificial means, have a professional do the job. Few things look worse than a bad coloring job on a man.

Even if you go to a pro, don't insist upon the hair shade of your blissful youth. When hair loses pigment, the skin gets paler at the same time. Too dark and dense artificial hair color announces itself and can make a fellow look older, not younger, because of the ghoulish contrast between skin and hair.

If you're not graying yet, think about what you'll want to do once the graying starts. And unless you're Dorian Gray, the odds are stacked that your hair will pale. Convinced you'll want to camouflage? At the first signs of graying, spring into action. Onlookers won't be shocked later by the sudden change that occurs when a very grayed fellow becomes colorful again.

And stay away from so-called "hair restorers" that you comb through your hair. They don't restore color, since they never invade the middle layer of the hair shaft where your own pigment is housed. Instead, they coat the shaft, and because they oxidize there, they can make hair rather brittle, more prone to breakage. Of course, if you condition your hair you dissipate this threat, but comb-through hair colorers also yield fairly unnatural-looking results. Sometimes, in combination with conditioners, they look even more unnatural.

If you have your hair professionally colored, chemicals will probably be involved. If so, your hair will be weakened, becoming progressively drier . . . unless you condition it even more scrupulously. In terms of working out, since salt goes after the hair too, when you color your hair you've got to treat it with even more compassionate kindness.

Oily hair almost never needs a conditioner, because the oil glands are ever busy, releasing oils the moment they can, usually making a conditioner superfluous. (Some conditioners are created for oily hair. They're less oily formulations. Necessary? Not often. Let your hair be your guide.)

Shampooing frequency ultimately depends upon conditioning frequency. Over the long haul, unless you have oily hair, it's smarter to shampoo and to condition often than to shampoo seldom without conditioning. With oily hair, frequent shampooing is still recommended, minus the conditioning.

DRESSINGS

Now, to qualify the remarks about conditioning.

For dry and normal hair, conditioning is invaluable. *Unless* you use one of the multitude of hair dressings that come in gels, creams, and liquids to control unmanageability and dullness. These products can supplant conditioners because they all do the same thing . . . *if* you prefer the look they impart. Not all of them are greasy kid stuff, and some are actually quite sophisticated. And quite expensive. But price is no guarantee of good results.

The only conceivable advantage of using a dressing instead of a conditioner is that you needn't shampoo before applying it. But it shouldn't be rubbed into dirty hair. On the other hand, you wouldn't want to use a conditioner *and* a dressing, because your hair would become sticky and gleam unnaturally.

SPRAYS

Hair sprays are supposed to hold your hair in place. The better they do that, despite what the commercials say, the stiffer or tackier (sometimes both) your hair feels to the touch. Overuse of sprays can make dry hair brittle. What's wrong with hair stirring in the breeze? Is it really a Herculean task to carry a comb?

BLOW DRYERS

The blow-dryer controversy is similar to the shampoo controversy. Directing lots of hot air at your scalp is not good . . . but the potential harm need not materialize: Blow drying can be as safe as shampooing-and-conditioning when precautions

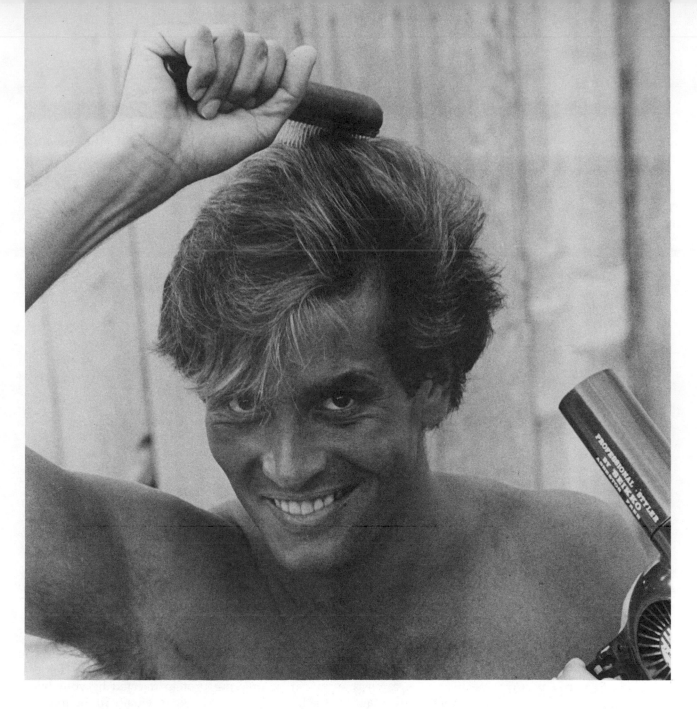

are taken. The main thing about the mane thing is not to horse around.

The first precaution: Since hair is most vulnerable when wet, rinse completely after shampooing and blot out the excess moisture with a terry towel. (This also makes blow drying go faster.)

The second precaution: Before wielding the dryer, spray your hair with a product specially formulated to coat the hair shafts and protect them against the heat. (If you've just conditioned your hair, this probably isn't necessary unless you have very dry hair.)

The third precaution: Don't release hot air against the tender scalp. Never set the dryer at its highest setting. Direct the airflow over and through the hair.

Too much dryer heat is too drying for dry and normal hair. Perversely, drying oily hair at the high setting won't dry up excess oil. Easily stimulated oil glands become even more stimulated by heat, so the scalp sends out more oil when the high setting is employed, compounding the oily-hair problem.

Of course, if you wear your hair in a short style, you'll never need a blow dryer. Just shampoo and rinse, condition as necessary, blot the hair as dry as possible, comb it into place, and let nature take its course.

CHAPTER 10

PORE BOY

BIG SPLASH

Do you really need this book to tell you men's and women's bodies aren't alike?

Not so obviously evident is the difference between male and female skin. A man's is slightly thicker, consequently slightly more resistant to wrinkling than a woman's. However, many a fellow, done in by his own machismo, is careless about skin care, losing his innate advantage through abuse. Don't.

Left unprotected from the elements, facial skin is bound to wrinkle. Wrinkling is primarily the result of age (which you can do nothing about) and dehydration (which you can do a lot about). Weather extremes, both hot and cold, rob the skin of moisture like bandits.

To look younger, fight wrinkles by fighting dehydration.

Unfortunately, the profuse sweating accompanying arduous workouts can be a steady cause of dehydration *if* you leave your facial (and body) skin unattended after an exercise session.

Before we speed directly into guidelines for skin care, though, here's a short dissertation on skin structure to show you *why* moisturizers are a man's, as well as a woman's, good pal.

CELL BLOCKS

Time for more morbid news. Just as the hair you see atop your head (and anywhere else, for that matter) is unliving protein rejected by your body, the layer of facial skin you see daily in the mirror is dead stuff too. Fear not. Skin you can't see is alive and, hopefully, well.

Your skin is composed of two layers. The outer layer (*epidermis*) is a group of flattened, dead cells that protect the interior of your organism from harmful environmental substances. This layer is pretty resilient and waterproof, despite its defunct state. Body oils help hold it together, but even so it's constantly being rubbed, washed, or scaled away. And that's good. Otherwise you would be toting the hide of an elephant.

Deep in the epidermis is the unseen *basal cell layer* (also called the *basal membrane*) where new living cells are manufactured. They are pushed to the surface, expiring en route, as newer cells are formed.

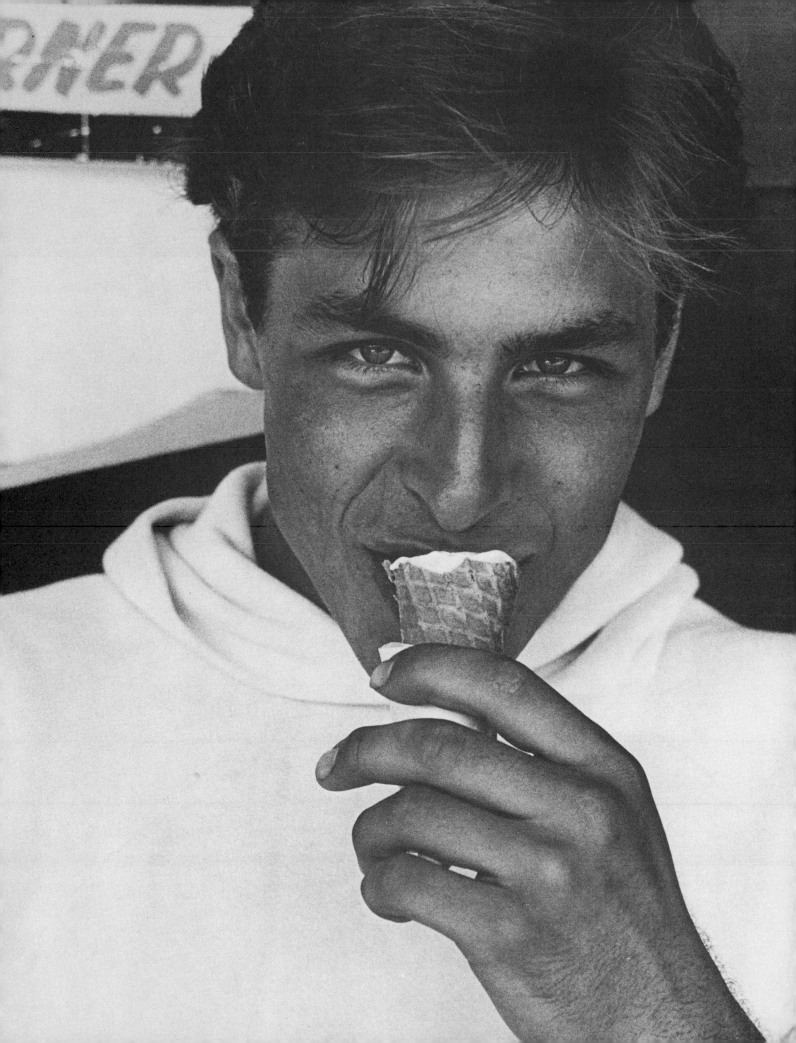

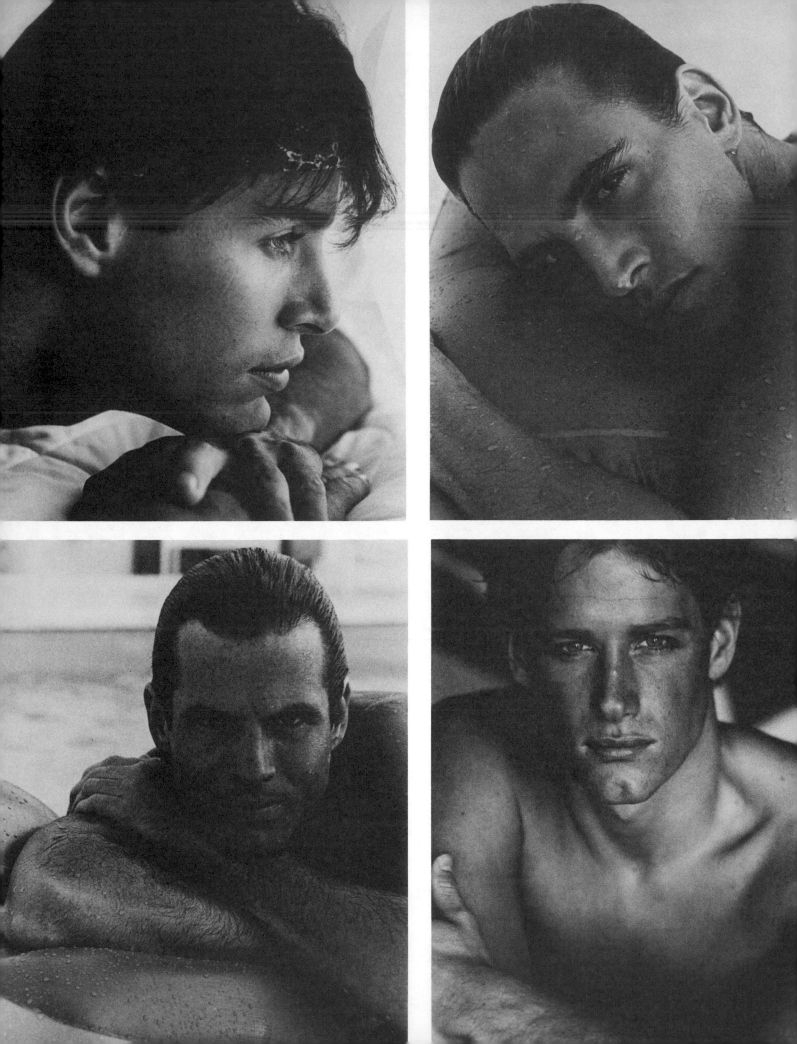

The migration—and the subsequent shedding—goes on and on.

Beneath the epidermis is the skin's innermost layer, the *dermis*. Its function is to support and feed the epidermis. But unlike the epidermis, which is constantly regenerating, the dermis can't reproduce itself. If it's injured, a permanent scar results.

Between the dermis and epidermis are connective fibers. When they break down or lose their elasticity, say hello to wrinkles. These fibers cannot regenerate themselves either, so "true" wrinkles—those caused by fiber breakdown, not "temporary" wrinkles caused by reversible skin dryness—are permanent additions to the topography of your face.

The dermis hosts a number of guests vital to body functions. Housed here are oil and sweat glands, plus hair follicles, all of which connect to the skin's surface via tubular ducts.

Just as the sebaceous glands lubricate hair shafts with oil (technically called *sebum*), these oil producers also secrete oil on the skin. When they pump out too much, the skin is oily. (That's why oily skin and oily hair are usually companions.) Too little, dry skin. Normal amounts, normal skin.

Sweat glands (the same kind as found on the scalp) regulate facial and body temperature too by producing perspiration to cool your face (and body).

The skin also has nerve endings to make you sensitive to heat, cold, pain, and touch. And it has deposits of melanin, which absorbs ultraviolet rays (tanning—or burning—the skin in the process) to guard internal organs against these dangerous rays.

Fundamentally, the skin acts as a shield. It's impervious to many substances that would be lethal if they penetrated the shield. Only water-based liquids are absorbed readily by the skin, and then only within the outer dead cells. Even so, if artificial steps aren't taken to "lock in" these watery substances, the moisture sucked up by the skin will simply evaporate.

WATER PROOF

Since unattended moisture evaporates from the skin, so-called moisturizers don't deserve the name. They don't add moisture to the face; they only entrap moisture—water—by sealing it in.

When the basal membrane is churning out new cells, initially they're plump little fellows, moist with water. But by the time they've reached your skin's surface, having lost almost all the water they started out with, they're thinnish and flattish. No more water is available to them from the inside except as perspiration, which isn't equal to the job of moisturizing really dry dead cells. External help is called for.

If running water is around, you can just turn on the faucet, splash your face with handfuls of water, then seal in the water with a "moisturizer."

To work, a moisturizer must contain a substance with which water can't mix—either oil or cream. Sebum is oily, so usually it helps hold in moisture. To some degree, it also holds water out. That's why you should wash your face to remove some of the sebum before moisturizing, making it easier for water to penetrate the epidermis.

If you have dry skin, you need extra help and an extra-high concentration of oil or cream in the moisturizer. (But not so much that you look like a greased pig after moisturizing.) If you have normal skin, you will gravitate toward a lighter-in-oil formulation. (Touch tells you how much oil a product contains. If it's very slippery, oil is plentiful.) If you have oily skin, you may never need a moisturizer, except for those times when the sun, the cold, or howling winds succeed in ridding your face of moisture despite your naturally oily shield.

When should you moisturize? With dry skin, anytime you wash your face, since washing away grime also washes away the little protective sebum you produce. (Since you probably can't moisturize that often, do so at least twice a day.) With normal skin, generally you can safely get by moisturizing once a day if you schedule it right. But if your skin becomes too dry—flakiness is a sure indication—moisturize twice. Oily skin? As noted, maybe you can skip moisturizing altogether.

Moisturizing after working out makes sense. During exercise, your face loses large amounts of moisture. And since you should always cleanse your face (body too) after a vigorous workout, soap effectively removes your natural moisture barrier. Not to mention dirt and sweat expelled from the pores.

If you exercise first thing in the morning, it's pointless to moisturize prior to the workout. Your perspiration would rapidly wash it away, and that's a waste of effort and product.

If you exercise at midday, with normal skin, see how your skin responds if you moisturize only once a day after working out. (If you shave in the morning, instead of moisturizing then, consider concluding the battle of the blade with an "after-shave" soother, a product remarkably similar to moisturizers. See the next chapter, Shaving Graces.)

With dry skin and a midday exercise schedule, moisturize morning and evening, plus after working out.

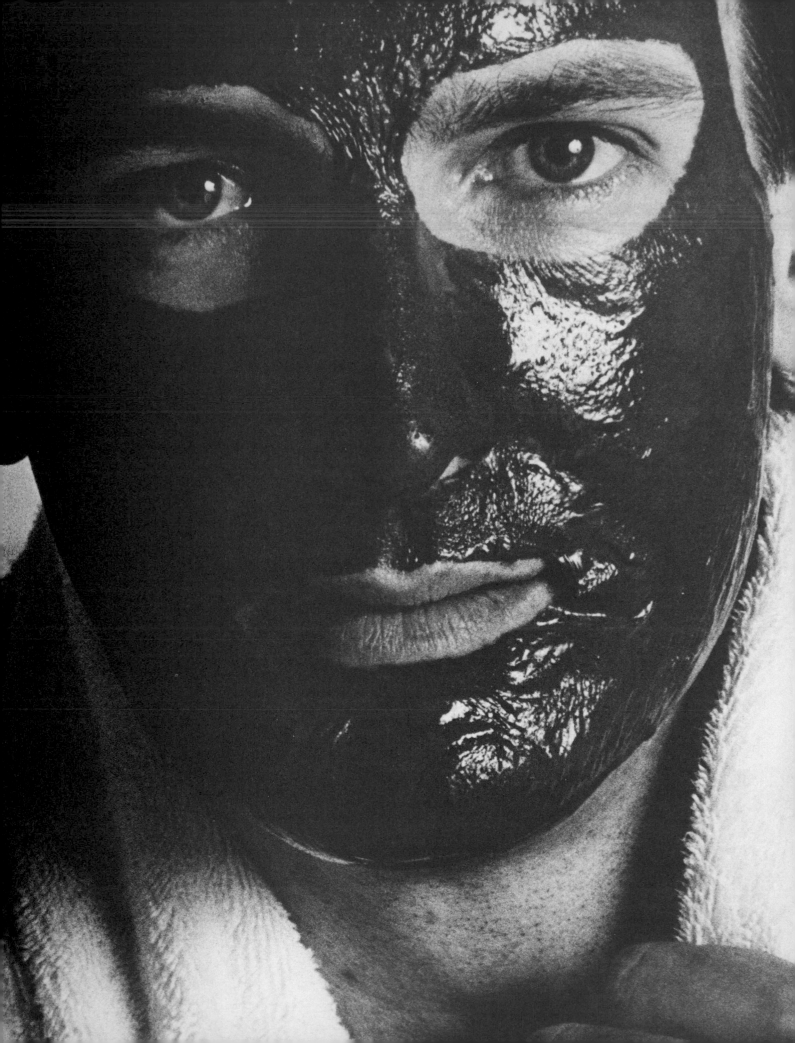

FACIALS

Many skin-care emporiums now claim a high percentage of male customers. Apparently men enjoy pampering just as much as women. And pampering is what facials have most to offer. Reputedly designed for deep pore cleansing, facials should never be considered more than an adjunct to your own skin routine. Even if you have a facial every week, you must wash yourself between visits.

Sifting through all the fluff, the benefits of facials stem more from the relaxation than from the cleansing. The massage, the spreading of creams, the wiping away of care—these steps in the facial satisfy the touch hunger that is many men's craving. Do they also offer a long-term healthful reward? Not if correct at-home procedures aren't subscribed to.

If men were less touchy about touching and being touched by their acquaintances, they wouldn't have to turn to strangers. Of course, women have facials too, but primarily because they think their skin condition will improve, *not* simply because they're seeking relaxation or a satiation of touch hunger.

One thing is sure. Facials, performed by caring professional fingers, feel *good*.

If you exercise in the evening, with either normal or dry skin, moisturize in the morning and after working out.

With oily skin, whenever you exercise, always treat your face to abundant splashes of water afterward.

In fact, to get the best out of moisturizing, always spend about half a minute cupping handful after handful of water onto your face before spreading a moisturizer *lightly* over your entire face and neck. (Globs of gooey moisturizer could clog pores and are counterproductive. A *thin* layer is all your skin needs and wants.)

CLEAN LIVING

Moisturizing is important, but don't ignore good ol' cleanliness. Without washing, even nonexercisers lack fresh faces. After all, more than any other body part (unless you're a nudist), the face is constantly exposed and constantly attracting airborne debris and pollutants. Oily skin holds tenaciously on to these pests. Pesty too are decomposed cells, sweat, waste, and other assorted transients on the face.

Facial cleansing is a necessity, but not slapdash cleansing. Despite the constant exposure, facial skin is relatively tender, while body skin is hardier. With any skin sensitivity (which invariably accompanies dry skin), use a facial soap, not a body bar, because the latter is just too strong for the face—especially a deodorant soap, developed for the body and not the face. (Body odor never emanates from the face, so deodorant soaps are doubly inappropriate for the face. Make that triply risky. See Gland Tidings, Chapter 13.)

After washing your face, splash it with lots of water to remove any suds from the pores.

If a man never experiences clogged pores, he'll probably never sport a whitehead or blackhead. Surprisingly, skin flare-ups are almost never the result of uncleanliness, although dirty skin can aggravate the situation.

Skin eruptions originate below the skin, not on top of it. When the pores are plugged, the sebum produced in the oil glands no longer has a natural escape route to the skin's surface. Imprisoned sebum just lolls around while the gland produces more of the substance.

At first the sebum remains colorless; the "plug" within the pore is then a whitehead. With time, the plug oxidizes and turns dark, into a blackhead.

And the oil glands keep churning out oil which remains trapped beneath the plug. The area becomes inflamed. If the oil still can't get out, a rupture occurs beneath the skin's surface, and inflammation is turned into infection.

Friend, keep those pores open.

One way pores clog is when dead surface cells

ANTIWRINKLE CREAMS

Most commercially available creams purporting to eliminate wrinkles really only hide them for a while. By hydrating the skin surrounding the wrinkles, they seem to make the lines disappear; you're wrinkle-free—until the moisture evaporates, and then the crevices are visible again.

Other wrinkle creams also operate on this shaky theory that what you don't see for a while disappears. These products *irritate* the skin's surface, causing it to swell up slightly. When the skin is swollen, the wrinkles aren't nearly as evident. But a swollen face does look puffy.

Nothing will truly get rid of wrinkles other than cosmetic surgery.

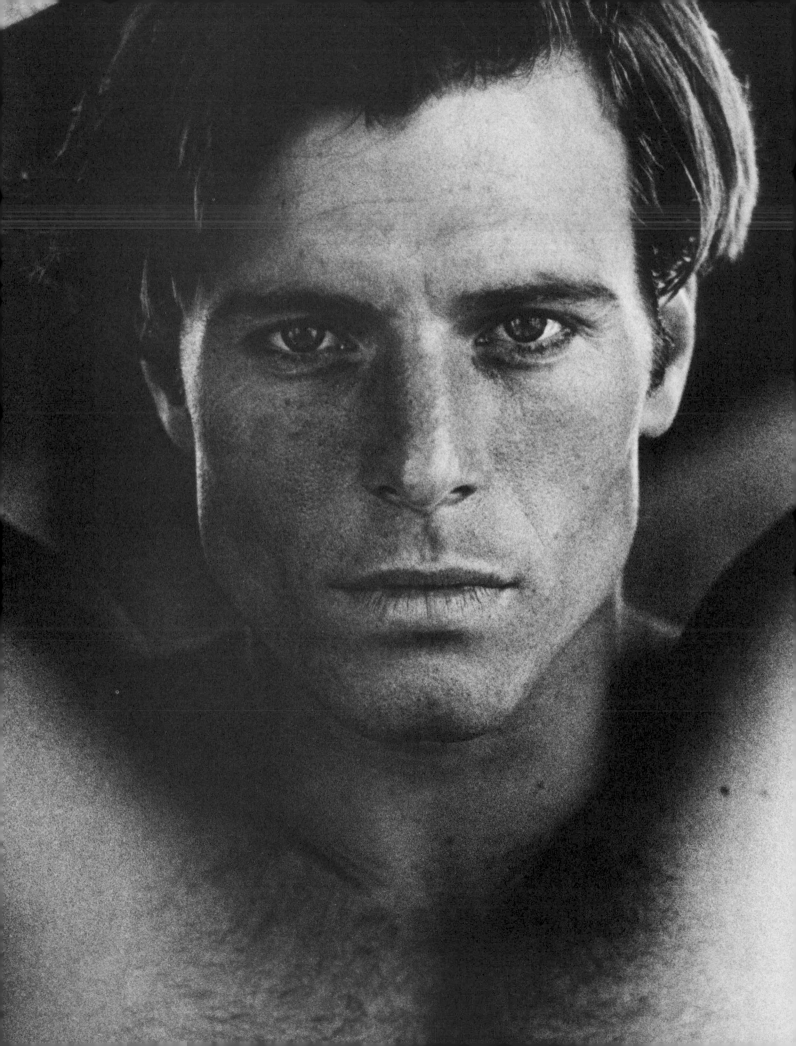

BRONZERS

An ongoing debate centers on whether bronzers—"tans from a tube"—are or aren't makeup. These harmless dyes (not to be confused with products that chemically alter your skin tone so the color can't be washed away) give you a ruddy complexion without basking in the sun. At night, in the privacy of your bathroom, you should bid the color a fond farewell. Without removing a bronzer before retiring, you'll smear it on your—or someone else's—pillowcase.

Because bronzers involve color, some debaters insist they're makeup. The opposition (perhaps composed of bronzer users) retorts that the color deposited by bronzers isn't opaque. It won't hide skin eruptions, for example; bronzers just give you and everything else they touch (including shirt collars) a deeper, bronzier hue.

If bronzers are applied sensibly and the pores remain unclogged, they're never injurious. (For a smoother application, if the product isn't termed a "moisturizing bronzer," it's best to spread on a moisturizer before spreading on the bronzer.) When applied with subtlety, they can compensate for a sallow complexion. Artlessly applied, they can look like clown's greasepaint.

Prejudicial thinking purports that *real men* never dabble with moisturizers or bronzers. That prejudice, like every form of small-minded bigotry, is something *real individuals*, male or female, pay no heed to. *Secure people* establish their own guidelines, in mind as well as appearance, without resorting to archaic sexual stereotypes and role-playing.

So what about wearing out-and-out makeup? It takes a hell of a lot of guts and an iconoclastic nature. Sexual double standards do still exist. But if you're convinced you'll make a better appearance wearing makeup, the more power—and makeup—to you. Newscasters do put on a cosmetic base (Pan-Cake is one tradename) before sitting on their anchor. But that's an example of another double standard. Logic and empathy do not rule the world. Nor the airwaves.

aren't sloughed. (This is a particular problem of men with oily skin, because the oils can bind dead cells.) If dead cells aren't shed, the skin's outer layer gets thicker and thicker, and the pore openings get smaller and smaller until they're practically nonexistent. The skin looks leathery, and skin tone is dull. The likelihood of flare-ups also increases.

THE SUN

The sun's burning rays attack the fibers connecting the dermis and epidermis, undermining their ability to support the skin. When these fibers are damaged or destroyed, they lose their elasticity and the skin loses its. In a sense, the skin "collapses" to fill the area where the healthy fibers once were. Since the fibers can't regenerate themselves, the skin remains in its collapsed state, and wrinkles map the face.

Positively no question exists about the sun's harmful effect on the skin. A suntan may look good, but looking ahead, never bathe yourself in sun without the protection of a sunscreen.

If you have a problem with literally thick skin, check out "scrubs"—granular soaps that thin the skin by abrading it to encourage the skin to shed its top layer more quickly. But beware of tender areas, such as under the eyes, that shouldn't receive this rough treatment.

Thick skin usually builds up wherever oil glands are densely populated. The forehead and the crevices around the nostrils are two such places. These areas are particularly problematic for guys with oily skin, and sometimes for fellows with normal skin. Scrub away with scrubs or, more inexpensively, with a coarse washcloth.

Astringents—usually alcohol-based liquids—also cut through greasy sebum to cleanse the pores. Alcohol is a chief ingredient in after-shave lotions, so splashing on an after-shave, then wiping the face—especially the nose and forehead—with cotton balls gets rid of excess oils and leaves you fragrant.

When should you follow these face-saving procedures? When necessary, *if* necessary. But don't use a scrub or an astringent immediately after working out. Your facial skin is already slightly irritated from all your sweating. Give it a break. Zonk it hours after or before working out.

CHAPTER 11

SHAVING GRACES

EDGE WISE

Only masochists get excited by the prospect of shaving. If it can't be fun, at least the battle of the blade shouldn't be skin-razing.

A secondary sexual characteristic that sprouts only after puberty, facial whiskers are usually coarser than the hair atop your head. Otherwise they too are waste protein. Although depilatories will eat them away, only one substance will safely but dramatically lessen their tensile strength—hot water. If you put on aerosol foam without first wetting the beard and then commence to shave, ouch!

Just as moisturizers don't literally moisturize, shaving preparations don't literally prepare the face for a blade shave. The more water you splash on your face before moisturizing, the more moisture you entrap; the longer you splash on *hot* water (just this side of scalding), the softer the beard becomes. If you splash for a minute or two before applying the shaving foam, then the foam becomes a shaving preparation.

Once the beard is wet, shaving foams and lathers keep it wet and keep it weak, so whiskers put up less of a fight when swiped by a sharp blade.

Water also swells the size of the whiskers. Shaving preparations do the same, surrounding and supporting the facial hairs so that they're plumper, easier targets to attack.

Foams and lathers also contain lubricating ingredients to promote razor glide. Cheap shaving preparations often dry up too quickly and are miserly with their lubricants. But shelling out for a high-priced spread doesn't guarantee you're getting your money's worth.

If a preparation is first-rate and the blade is the best, and if you allow yourself some extra time for self-preservation, shaving needn't be torture. Here is war counsel for winning the battle of the blade.

Set the scene with a steamy shower or bath. Without any help from you, the heated steam will start softening your beard.

Use your hands and head. Dousing your whiskers for a full minute or two with handfuls of hot water is the surest way to lower their resistance.

Save face with a rich shave foam. Extra lubrication makes for smoother gliding.

Be edgy. A dull razor blade can sabotage all your preliminary tactics. Time-abused cutting edges pull at the beard and leave a ragged stubble behind. They're also more likely to nick and tear the skin. Keeping the blade wet and clean also makes shaving less of a pain.

Plot your defenses. It's better to shave safely twice a day than once rashly. Don't shave against

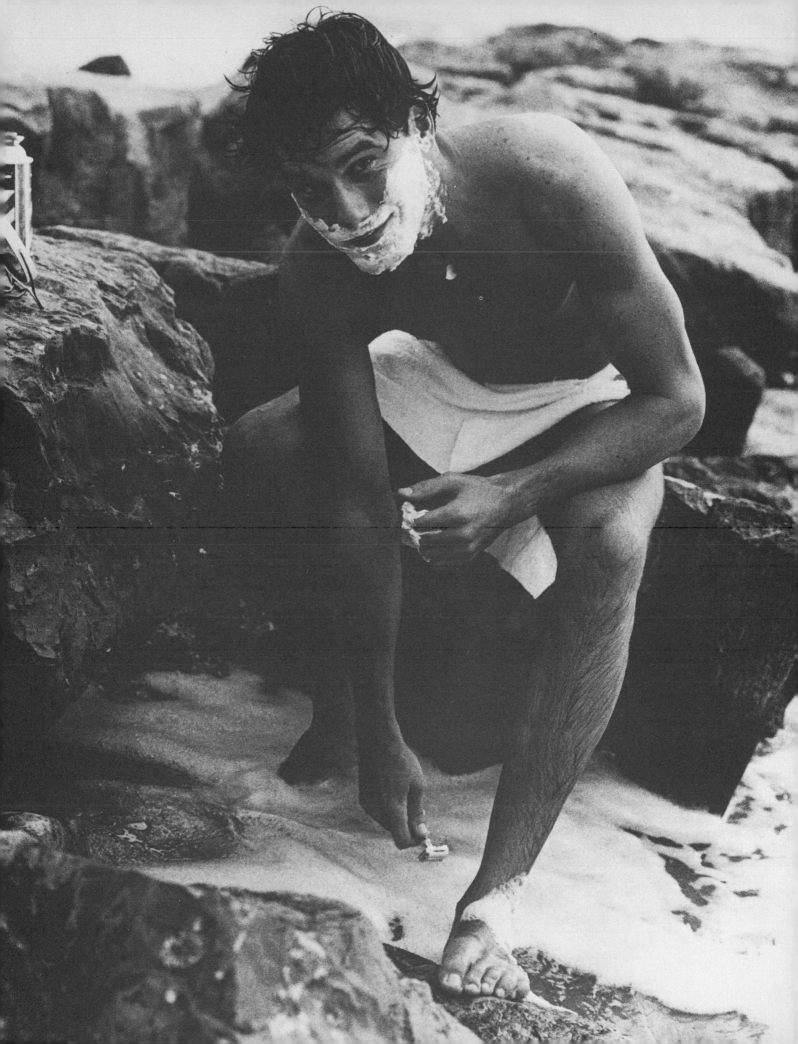

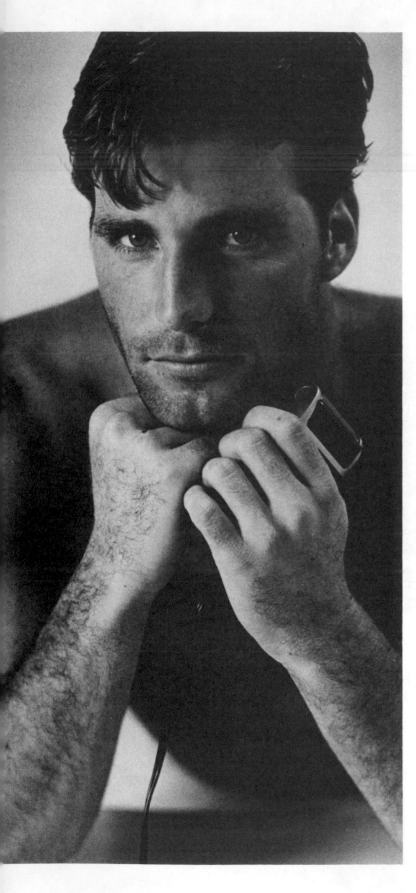

the grain on the misguided premise that you're getting a closer shave: Doing so increases the odds you'll develop ingrown hairs and prickly irritations.

Map out your strategy. The chin and upper lip sport the coarsest beard hairs. Shaving there last allows maximum softening by the water and foam.

Stay sharp. After shaving, rinse the blade with a steady flow of water. Don't dull it by wiping with a tissue or towel.

Spare yourself. Shaving foams are drying. Resort to friendly water to rinse all residue away.

ROUND & ROUND

Strategies for a safe shave are diametrically opposed if you use an electric razor. Instead of trying to weaken the beard with water, you first seek to strengthen it with a pre–electric-shave preparation. If you lowered its resistance, a whisker might be supple enough to bend when encountering the rotary blades of an electric shaver, escaping totally instead of falling.

On the other hand, you still want to lubricate your face, because razor burn is no fun.

The first step in electric shaving is washing the face with soap and water. But since the stiffest whiskers are the driest whiskers, you next splash on the pre–electric-shave preparation. Among its ingredients are alcohol, noted for its drying capabilities. It also degreases the beard, making it more rigid still.

Likewise among the ingredients are lubricating oils deposited on the skin so that the shaver will glide, not lurch.

Now the whiskers are standing tall, waiting to be lopped, and your skin is slick enough for the electric razor to travel its contours smoothly.

When you've finished shaving, your skin will still feel slick. Soap and water—lots of water—should remove any remnants of the pre–electric-shave preparation. If they don't, cotton balls soaked in alcohol or witch hazel (which carries less of a sting) and wiped across the shaved zone should.

SLAP DASH

Whichever shaving method you employ—blade or electric razor—your skin is more sensitive afterward. For one thing, it's drier, because protective oils have been scraped away during the dewhiskering. Also removed is part of the epidermis' top layer. Although you try to be gentle, the skin is abraded. Even if you can't see them, there are superficial nips and cuts.

Unless your skin is especially dry or sensitive, disinfecting it with a splash of after-shave can't really hurt, although it might sting. Colognes, even heavier in alcohol concentration than after-shaves, will give your face a harder slap without spreading around the healing ingredients formulated in after-shaves. (Unless the cologne is touted as an after-shave cologne; even so, to carry more fragrance than conventional after-shaves, colognes are always heavier in alcohol). Astringents and pure alcohol are antiseptics, but they sting more than either after-shaves or colognes.

You don't need to slap your face to bring a shave to a satisfactory conclusion. A new generation of after-shave products—called after-shave balms, conditioners, and soothers and by assorted other names—cut down on the alcohol and inject emollients and lubricants in its stead. Some are fragranced, some aren't.

To avoid getting stung, you'll find balms an excellent alternative to after-shave lotions . . . unless you have oily skin. (Oily skin, you've noticed, always calls for exceptional treatment.) Most balms are enriched with oils or creams, so thay have no place on oily skin. A very few, however, come in the liquid consistency of after-shaves, and they're acceptable for all skin types.

To get the most out of a balm after shaving, rinse your face with lots of water, then apply the balm. Most such products will seal the face the same way self-proclaimed moisturizers do.

BEYOND THE FRINGE

Knowing the right way to shave—and to end a shave—isn't tantamount to knowing when to do it.

Unfortunately, there's no good way to integrate shaving and workout sessions. If you shave immediately before working out, sweat will wash away any soother you applied to your skin after shaving. The salt in the sweat may cause the microabrasions to sting. Pores will open wider during exercise as perspiration gushes through them, increasing the possibility (though hardly the probability) of irritation, even rashes.

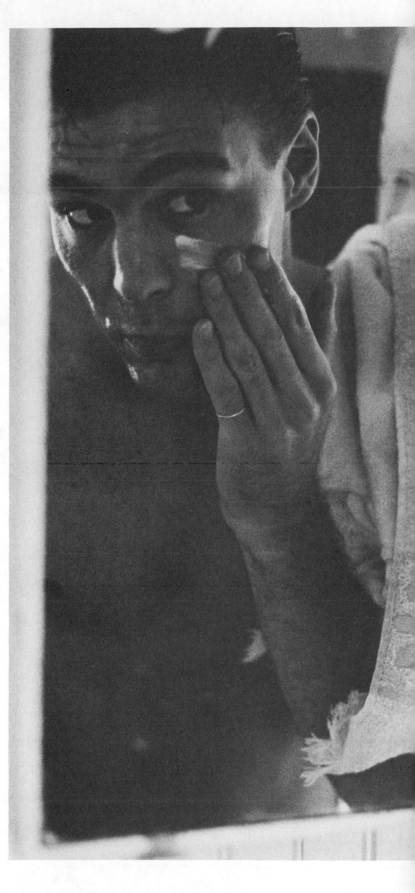

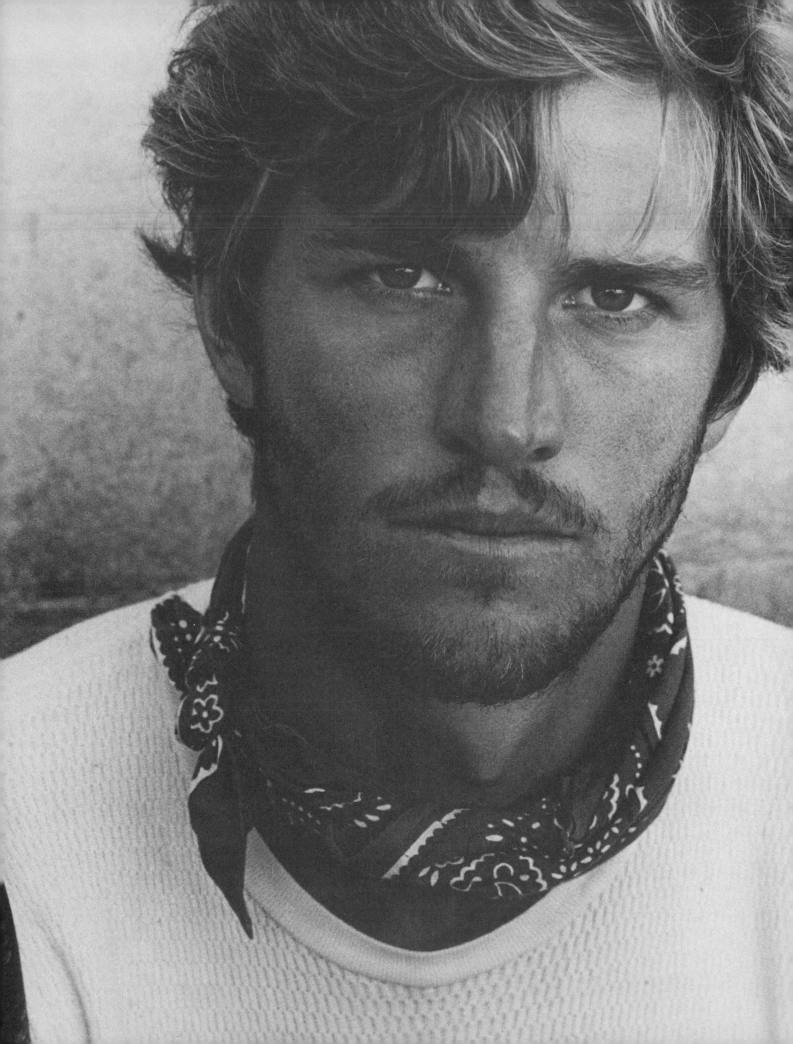

On the other hand, if you don't shave before working out, your stubble might chafe and feel uncomfortable when you execute the movements that require tucking your chin against your chest.

If you shave immediately after working out, capillaries on the surface of your face will be relatively engorged because of your exertion. It's easier to nick yourself and harder to stop the blood from flowing. Also, the sweat bath from working out is automatically irritating to the face, so shaving will doubly prove an irritant.

What's the answer? No truly satisfactory one unless your whiskers are very cooperative. If your beard is light, for example, you can probably shave once a day whenever you feel like it without threat of a five-o'clock shadow. But if your facial hair is pushier than that, most likely you must shave before heading off to work. If you exercise before trudging off to bring home the bacon, toss a coin to decide whether to shave before or after exercising. As a time saver, shaving after working out is more logical because you can consolidate most of your grooming regimen within one span after the exercise.

If you work out midday or evening, shave in the morning and feel fortunate.

BEARDS

Your chin is under your beard (if you've grown one), as is facial skin. Whether hidden or not, your face needs washing. So does a beard. Facial soap should suffice for both, but treat your face tenderly. Don't attempt to use a coarse beard as a washcloth. Get your fingertips between your whiskers against flesh, then gently rotate them to work up a lather. Rinse with lots of water. Flakes in a beard are almost never dandruff; they're usually residual soap that hasn't been swept away.

Blotting a beard with a dry towel gets rid of most of the water. While your beard is still damp, carefully comb it with a wide-toothed comb before tangles set in. Never brush it while wet, because wet hair (especially coarse wet hair) breaks easily. Comb the beard in the direction in which you want it to lie. Blow dryers are *verboten* on beards.

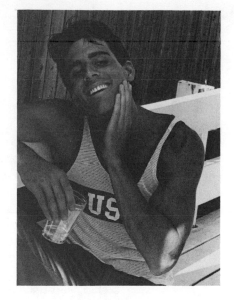

CHAPTER 12

LIQUID ASSETS

STALLED

Good grooming is little more than keeping clean, so it follows that a well-groomed body is necessarily a clean one. Colognes or deodorants can never take over for a steamy shower or a relaxing bath. Yet if you shower or bathe several times a day, rather than coming across as belonging to Mr. Clean, your body might instead rival Father Time's.

The lurking villain, per usual, is perspiration.

Per usual, the way your body functions helps you determine how to combat the problems inherent in going overboard in body cleansing.

From your reading about hair and skin care, you're aware that whenever you exercise vigorously you sweat a lot. Not only that, your perspiration whisks away protective oils, so when you're through working out, your body is at its most vulnerable. If you wash your body after exercising—

and you should, if only out of deference to your associates' noses—soapy action also conspires to leave your body unprotected. When you scrub your body spotlessly clean, rinse away the suds, and do nothing else, you're inviting dry, flaky skin from forehead to ankle. The harsher your soap, the more drying it can be.

To offset the drying capabilities of shampoo, you used a hair conditioner, which can be thought of as a hair moisturizer. To entrap moisture in your facial skin, you used a skin moisturizer. To trap moisture inside the rest of your surface, after showering or bathing, dry yourself halfheartedly. While you're still damp, spread a body moisturizer over your whole body. (Unless you have oily skin. In that case, you usually shouldn't use a body moisturizer.)

But what is a body moisturizer? Any type of lotion with enough oil or cream in its formulation so water can't sneak past its barrier. Baby oil, though sometimes too sticky to the touch, is an effective

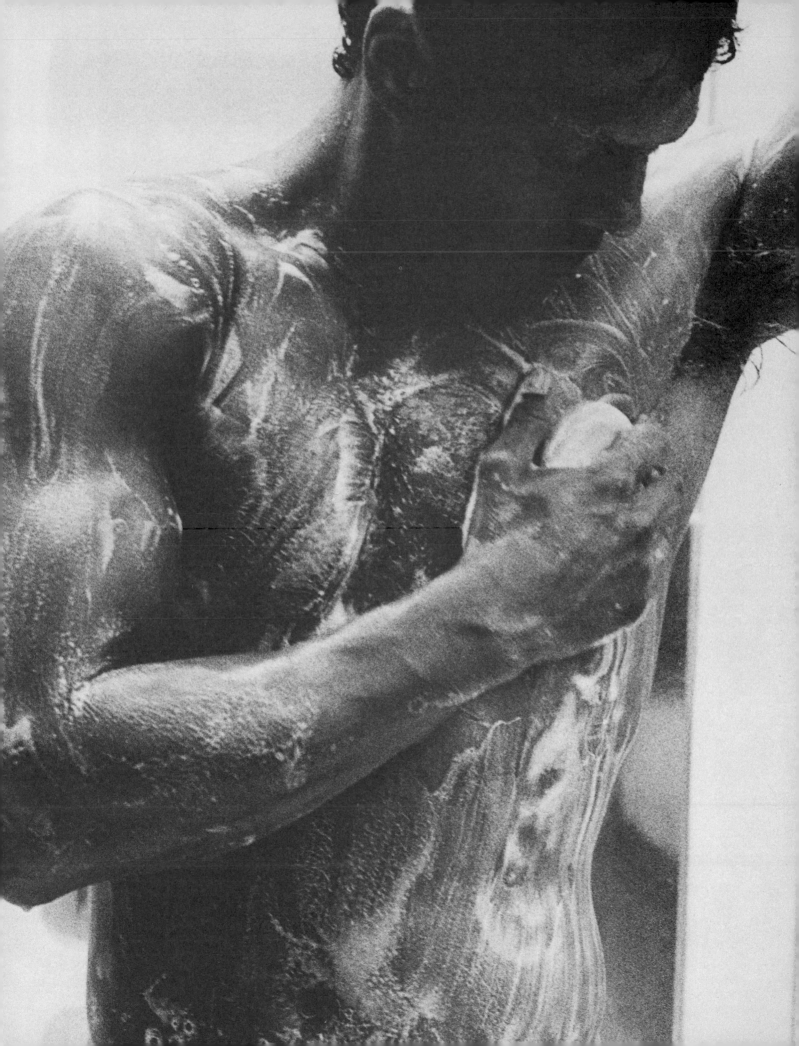

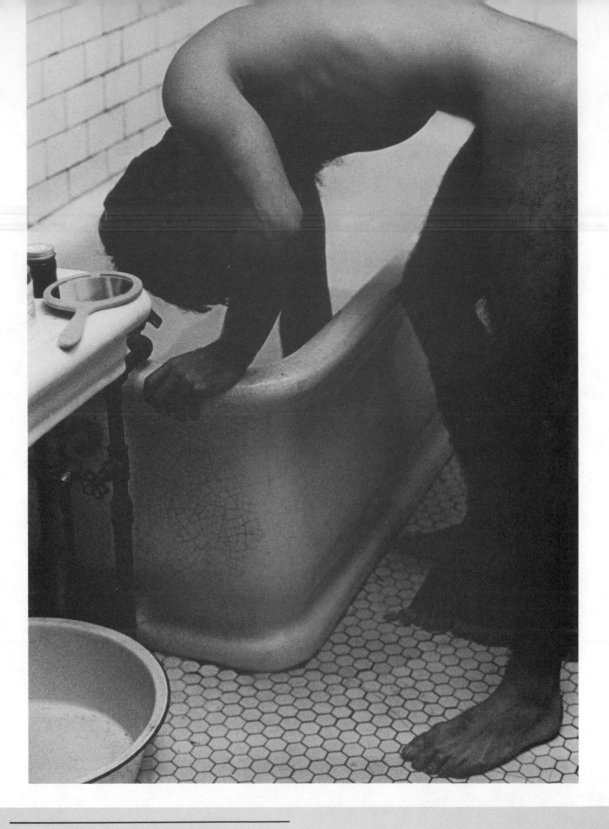

BODY SPLASHES

These are really little more than body colognes. In formulation, they're less concentrated with fragrance than facial colognes. Both are high in alcohol content (not the drinkable kind).

When alcohol is doused on a warm body, the effect is always cooling. The end result also tends to be drying.

If you find a body splash exhilarating, take your pleasure from the bottle. Following up the splash with a body moisturizer won't make you tingle, but doing so soothes and smooths roughed-up body skin.

COLD SHOWERS

Although cold showers have their time and place, immediately following a tough workout is certainly not the time. You must first cool your body down before immersing it in any water. The harder you exercise, the higher your internal temperature rises and the longer it takes you to cool down. To avoid any shock to your system, opt for a lukewarm shower or bath. If you crave the tingle of cold water, *gradually* increase the cold.

Speaking of cold. In cold weather, baths are supposedly more drying to the skin than showers. But if you add bath oil to the water—*not* bath bubbles—that blows the whole theory to smithereens. In fact, if you bathe with bath oils, they take the place of body moisturizers, so you can perform two grooming functions in the same place at the same time.

body moisturizer. So is petroleum jelly, although its gloppy consistency makes it more unappetizing as a body spread than baby oil. Most inexpensive skin-care lotions sold in discount drugstores perform as body moisturizers.

One thing a body moisturizer is not is an expensive facial moisturizer. Moisturizers for facial skin are buffered with extra emollient ingredients to soothe the face and to be more pleasing to the touch than cheaper general-purpose varieties. But this doesn't necessarily make the more costly ones any more efficient.

When should you moisturize your body? After exercising, of course, when you've showered or bathed. Once a day is enough, even for dry skin. With normal skin, there's relatively little risk if you moisturize your body only every other day or so. With oily skin, don't bother unless your skin suddenly becomes patchy. And then moisturize only the dry patches.

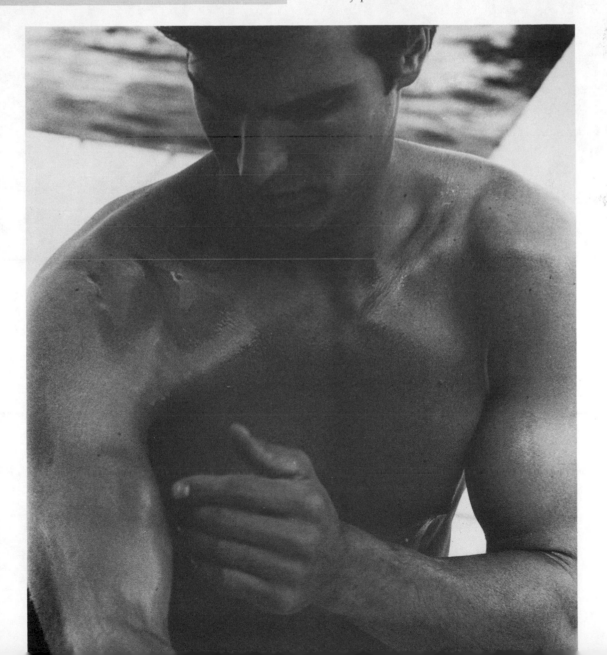

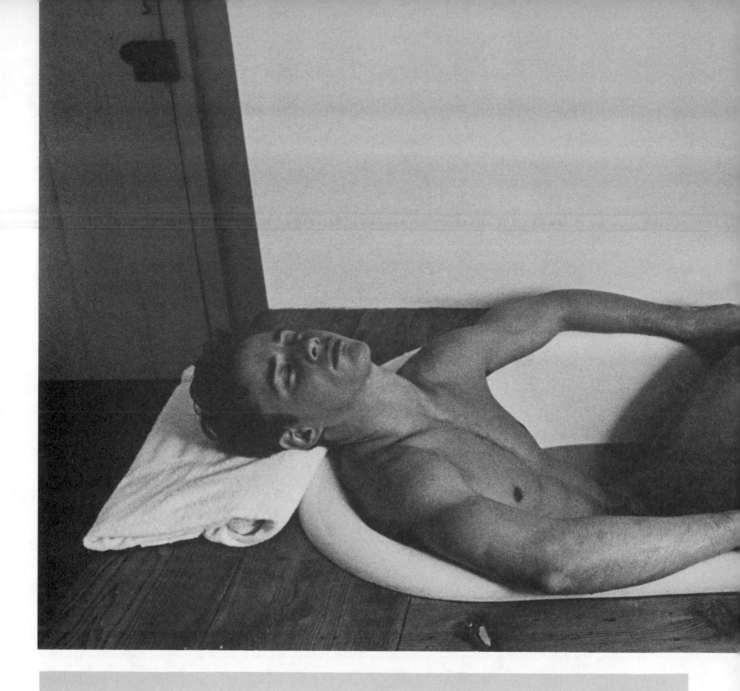

HEAT RASHES

The profuse sweating accompanying heavy work-outs can be very problematical, particularly among joggers who spend long periods of time inside sweaty sweat shirts. Tiny pustules on the back often result. Strictly speaking, these aren't heat rashes; they're perspiration rashes. Here's what happens.

Perspiration becomes trapped inside the hair follicle without proper release. The skin swells. The pressure inside the follicle causes it to erupt. Minor infection ensues. Minor becomes major if ignored.

One way to fight this phenomenon is to dry up the irritations as soon as they appear. Both strong soap and alcohol help. Moisturizers don't. In fact, at the first sight of these little buggers, steer clear of moisturizers.

Another way to fight this acnelike rash is to keep sweaty garments away from the skin and to shower as soon as possible after sweating it out. If showering must be postponed, rubbing the body with alcohol helps. Clogged pores always increase the potential for rashes.

Although body moisturizers are generally recommended, not so if you tend to break out in body rashes of any kind. On the other hand, if you've been exercising regularly and have never experienced difficulties with either rashes or skin dryness, leave well enough alone and don't start the moisturizing habit. Why meddle with success?

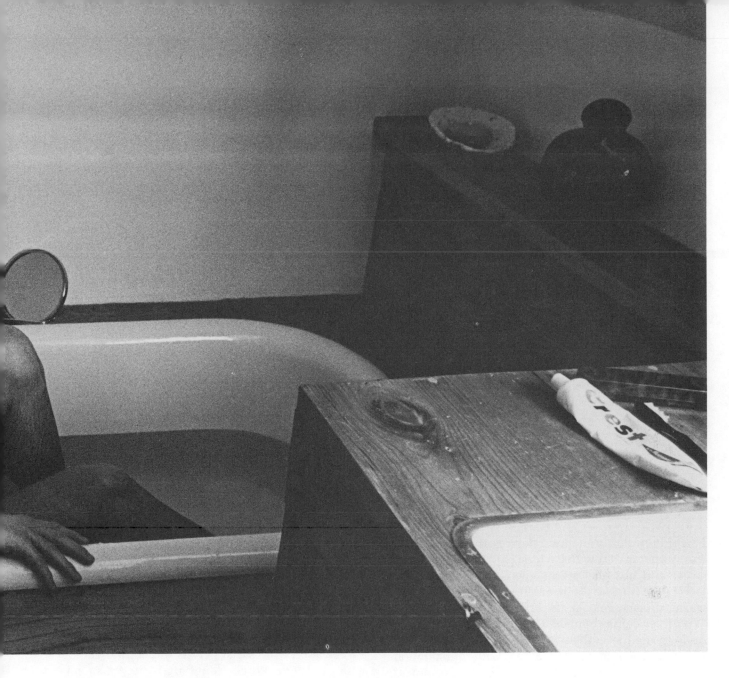

Is showering several times a day really bad for you? Yes, if your body skin has any inclination toward dryness. But not even then if you take moisturizing precautions.

If you work out first thing in the morning, it makes no sense to clean your body before exercising. If you don't work yourself into a fresh sweat, one cleansing—and one moisturizing, if that—after working out will normally suffice.

If you exercise at midday, you face that old decision of whether to cleanse your whole body once or twice a day. Judge for yourself. With oily skin, if you don't want to offend, twice is better, since you become rank more easily than a dry-skinned neighbor.

If you exercise in the evening, wouldn't you feel more secure throughout the day if you showered or bathed in the morning as well as after working out?

Depending upon your night life, you may choose to clean up before dozing off to dreamland.

CHAPTER 13

GLAND TIDINGS

ESP

Perspiration left to its own devices is usually odorless. Sweat mixed with bacteria isn't. Washing away sweat and dirt also spirits away bacteria breeding faster than bunnies on the skin, particularly in dark, warm, moist areas like the armpits.

With bacteria banished and sweat down the drain, gone too is the source of B.O. . . . until persevering bacteria return, along with perspiration . . . and the renewed prospect of B.O. Cleanliness helps keep you from smelling like a garbage heap, but it can't perform the task of total odor control unaided. To smell swell, add either deodorants (which simply mask unpleasant aromas) or antiperspirants (which reduce the amount of sweat released on the skin to help nip repugnant odor in the bud).

Understanding a little more about the mechanisms of B.O. will help you plot your strategy to resist falling prey to its sway.

GROSS PROFIT

Sweat glands cover the entire body, but they come in two kinds. The less offensive ones are called the *eccrine glands*, and they're also the most numerous, particularly on the forehead, palms, and soles.

Apocrine glands, though fewer in number, make up for their relative paucity by excreting more than the salty perspiration that the eccrine glands release. The apocrine variety, flourishing in the underarms and in the genital and anogenital areas as well as the navel and around the breasts, expel a sticky, whitish fluid laden with metabolic by-products.

Regulation of internal heat is the eccrine glands' main function. While doing that, they also join forces with sebum to keep the skin moist and to retard the premature shedding of the skin's cuticle layer. When it's very hot (or when you're working out at a hot trot), sweat drips off the skin, first in the areas of highest glandular concentration—the forehead, palms, and soles.

The apocrine glands are more interested in eliminating metabolic wastes, and they do a more fervent job when hepped up by heat or activity. Stress and physical excitation also turn them on.

Bacteria are most prolific where perspiration can't evaporate—including the same places where the apocrine glands abound. Although the apocrine glands don't release nearly as much fluid as the eccrine glands, when the milkier substance from the former commingles with the waterier substance from the latter, the apocrine secretions are mixed

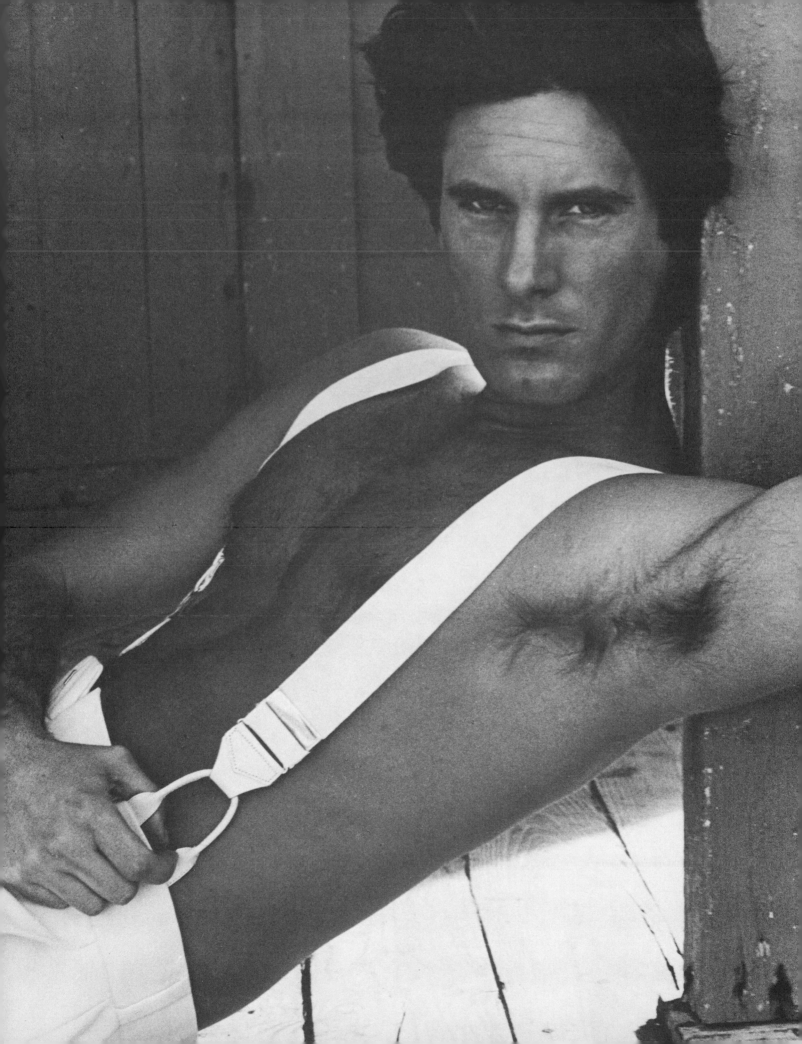

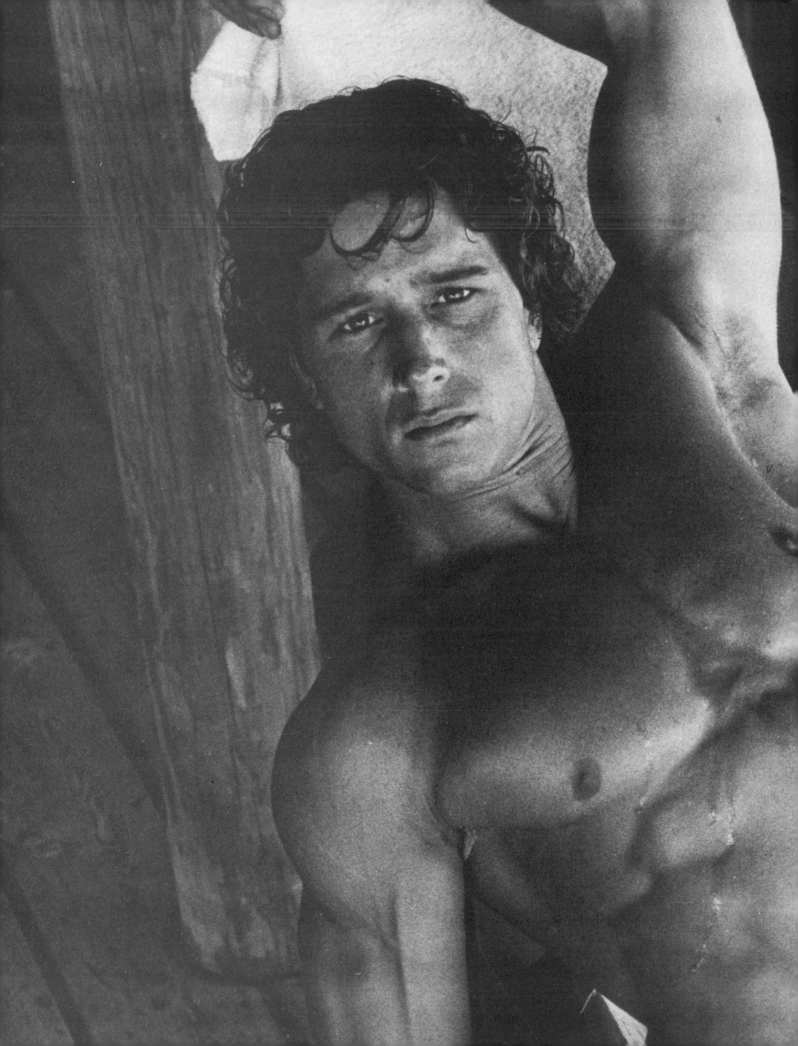

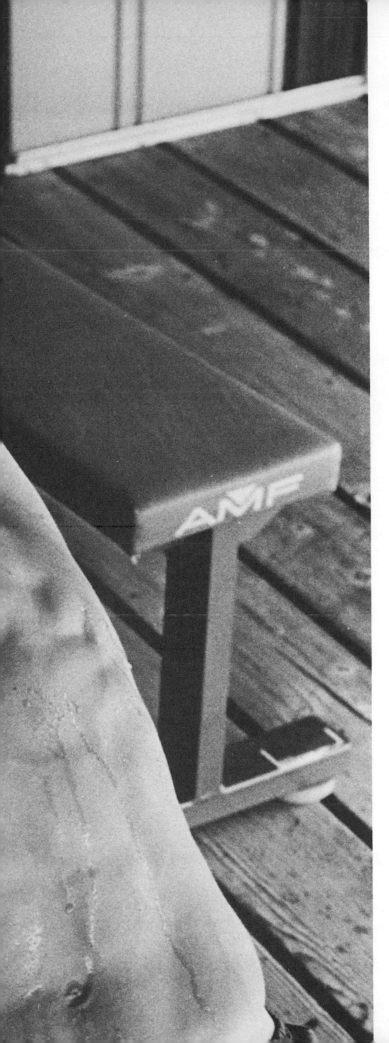

and spread, encountering more bacteria in the merger. Body odor is the expansive result of the conglomeration. The rankest odor is due to apocrine-gland excretions.

Since body odor wouldn't bloom so flagrantly in the absence of bacteria, however, removing bacteria removes the major source of body odor. (You wouldn't want to stop perspiring or you'd die.) And since soap and water removes these microorganisms for a time, to get a head start on odor control, start out with a clean body. Then be particularly painstaking about cleansing areas where apocrine glands are most populous.

SWEAT SHOP

The B.O. story underscores why deodorant soaps are not advisable for cleansing the face, where no apocrine glands are found. Because deodorant soaps are ruthless in removing sebum—their claim to fame for the body—they can even increase your likelihood of getting sunburned if you go out in the noonday sun unprotected after showering.

Antiperspirants don't stop all sweating, but they retard its output. For this reason, they're helpful *after* working out, but not before or during: You don't want to stem perspiration while exercising, because you don't want to collapse from heat prostration.

If you exercise solo and aren't sensitive to your animalism, forget about your armpits before working out. If you exercise in a group and don't exactly smell like a rose once you start steaming, douse on a body talc before getting under way. Talcs don't interfere with perspiration; their granules absorb perspiration (or some of it), keeping you drier and keeping the sticky stuff from spreading unrestrainedly.

While you're sprinkling that talc, give your crotch a dusting too, plus all other areas where apocrine glands lurk. Any fragranced product releases more aroma as your body heats, so don't select an overpowering or offensive talc.

For fragrance to be incorporated into any liquid product, alcohol is invariably present. So are fixatives. While seldom harmful in after-shaves or colognes, alcohol combined with other chemicals in deodorants and scented antiperspirants can be harsh enough to sting—a certain sign the skin is being superficially irritated. The irritation is cumulative, so repeated applications of a deodorant and/or antiperspirant throughout the day aren't satisfac-

COLOGNE

Cologne is neither an after-shave lotion nor a deodorant. It's a liquid to make you smell a way you don't, not to cover the way you do.

Even products advertised as "unscented" aren't odorless. The manufacturers try to eliminate any distinctive aroma within the essential ingredients with other, nonessential neutralizing ingredients to create an "unscented" smell.

Unless you are allergic to any of the ingredients, you shouldn't get hung up on the formulae for colognes or any other grooming products as long as you like the smell and like the products. However, fragrances affect each other.

Say you use a musky cologne. And say you wash your body with a foliage-scented deodorant soap. The two fragrances will combat, not complement, each other. If you roll on an unscented deodorant, its unscented scent could add new conflict.

One way to get around incompatible fragrances is to buy all your grooming aids from one company which infuses them all with the same scent. That can cost. Another way is to use only "unscented" products—unscented shampoo, unscented soap, unscented antiperspirant, et cetera—except for your cologne. Although the unscented ones aren't truly fragrance-free, at least they shouldn't constantly be struggling to upstage each other. With less intense aromas remaining in the background, cologne can assume the fragrance spotlight.

tory. Rashes can erupt. Should they occur, lay off the products immediately, and find gentler substitutes after the irritation clears up.

COMMON SCENTS

For all the reasons previously mentioned, it makes no sense to deodorize immediately before working out except for a sprinkle or two of talc. So when should you try to undermine B.O.?

If you exercise first thing in the A.M., easy timing. Work out, cool down, shower or bathe, then slap on that antiperspirant. (Although antiperspirants are no panacea for B.O., with conscientious cleansing they are a decided boost. If fragranced, they mask odor while outperforming deodorants by postponing part of the cause of that odor.)

However, if you cleanse your body in very hot water, you'll stimulate your sweat glands. Don't

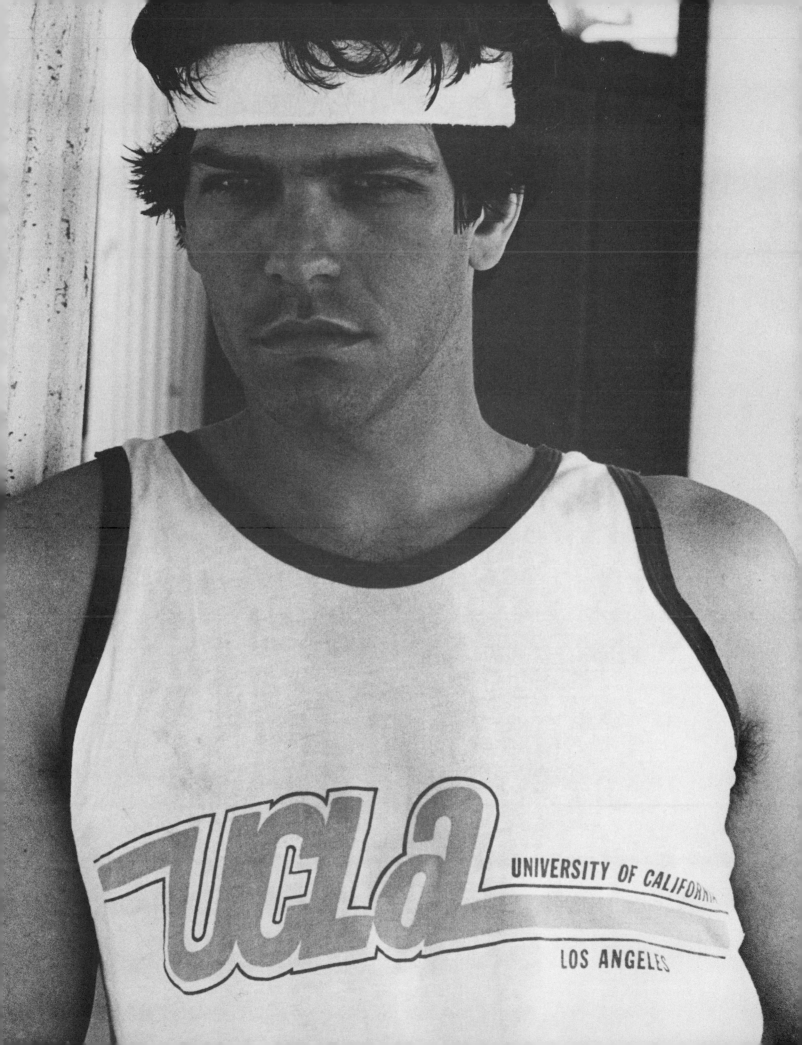

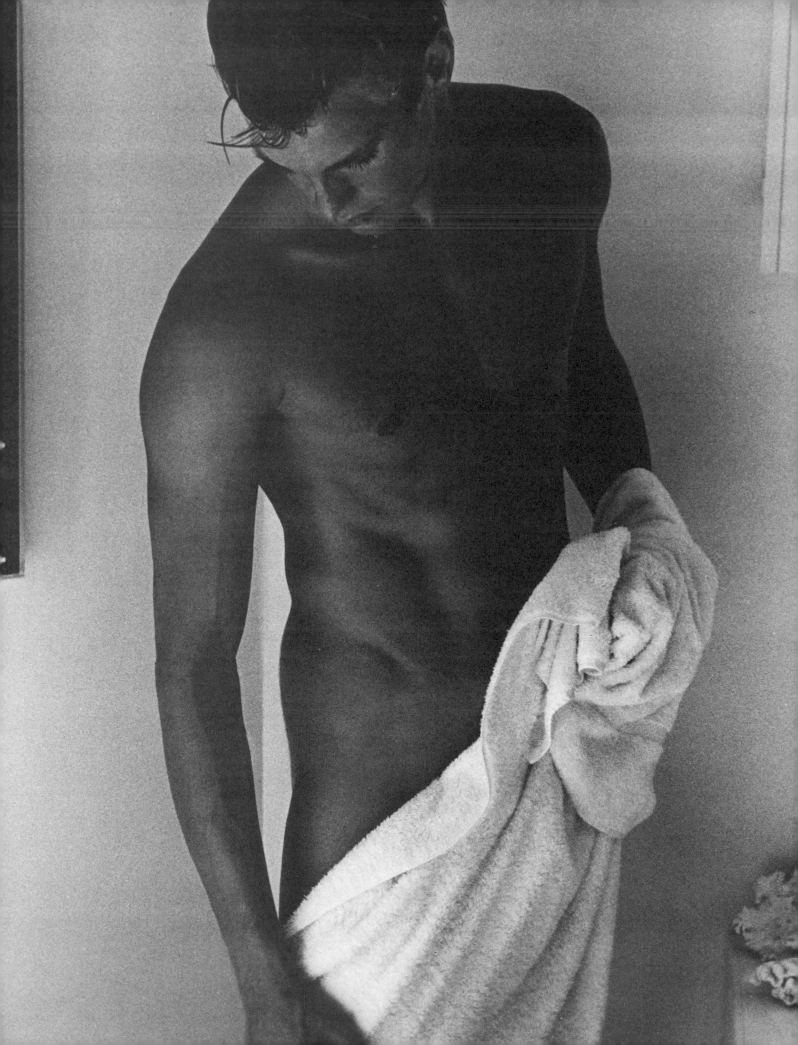

end your cleansing at full heat. Turn the water to lukewarm or cool, and rinse your sensitive areas at the reduced temperature. Don't towel them furiously to dry; that too gets the glands active again. Blot gently.

If you can, wait several minutes before putting on the antiperspirant. If you normally sweat heavily, follow it up with a dusting of body talc to absorb moisture (basically sweat) as it builds up again. Dust your crotch and chest too.

If you exercise midday or evening, and if you shower twice a day, wield the antiperspirant after your workout, and protect yourself following the other body cleansing with ample talc.

The crotch is too touchy a place for an antiperspirant. But it's also a hot spot. Tight, synthetic underwear unleashes the apocrine glands. So does a jock. Reach for the talc.

Clothing harbors both odor and bacteria. Talcs and antiperspirants do only so much. They can't do the laundry.

FIRM FOOTING

Apocrine glands aren't the villains in foot odor. Carelessness is. If you don't wash your feet scrupulously, dirt and dead matter are left between your toes to decompose. They don't need the assistance of apocrine glands to smell like hell. Moisture and bacteria are more than ready to take over.

While cleansing after working out, pay special attention to your feet. Foot powders are essentially talcs for the feet, just not so finely granulated. They make sense in combating unpleasant scents on your pedal extremities.

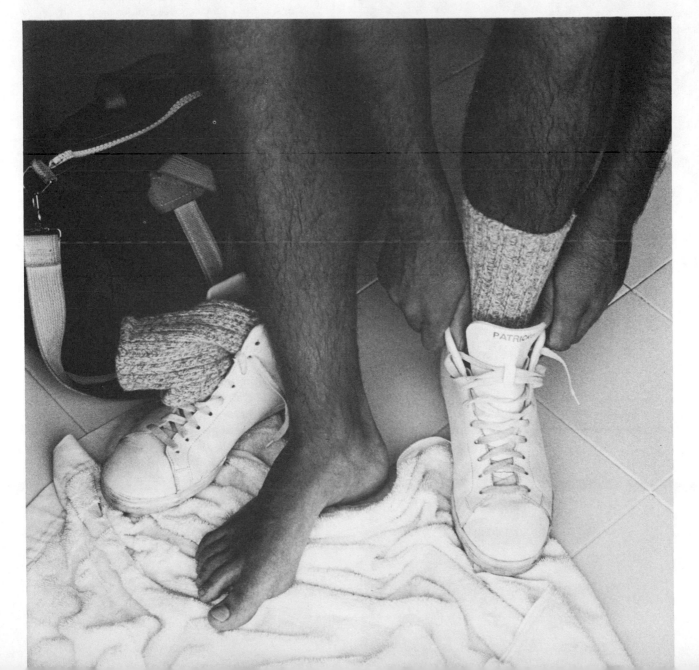

FOOTWEAR

In most cases while you're working out, bare feet will get you through (except for some of the aerobics), but if you want to wear shoes (and socks), wear the right kinds—which may be different depending upon your activities.

You should never jog barefoot or in your dress oxfords, because your feet and legs would not be protected against injury. A good jogging or running shoe should be lightweight enough so your feet and legs don't drag, and the soles must be cushioned enough to absorb the shock of pounding the pavement without transmitting the trauma to your feet. A rolling sole at the heel also helps. Some padding at the back of the shoe protects the Achilles tendon from jolts. Padded arch supports keep feet stable and offset their tendency to incline inward.

You wouldn't play tennis barefoot or in your oxfords either. But neither should you wear running shoes. Tennis demands more twisting of the feet than running, so to facilitate the stop/start, multidimensional movement, lace up tennis shoes—which, being somewhat squarer and heavier than running shoes, don't offer the same kind of support as those designed for running.

Shoes for racquetball have an additional requirement atop those for tennis: The soles must have rounded edges for climbing the walls.

To be on a firm footing when working out, go to the best shoe store around and seek the help of a knowledgeable salesperson. Spring for the best you can afford. Once again, aesthetics are secondary to function.

If you wear athletic shoes with casual—not sports —attire, running shoes are the all-around excellent choice.

Truthfully, to be really conscientious, you should wash your feet twice a day, but unless you shower twice daily, you probably won't. Nor is it likely that you'll wash them in warm water with soap, rinse them in cold water, dry them carefully—especially between the toes—rub them with alcohol-soaked cotton balls, wait until they're thoroughly dry again, and then douse them with a foot powder. That's the best way to cleanse feet, but it is a drag.

If you ever have an unfortunate encounter with athlete's foot that over-the-counter remedies don't remedy, don't procrastinate. See a doctor. Virulent athlete's foot can infect the soles and under the toenails.

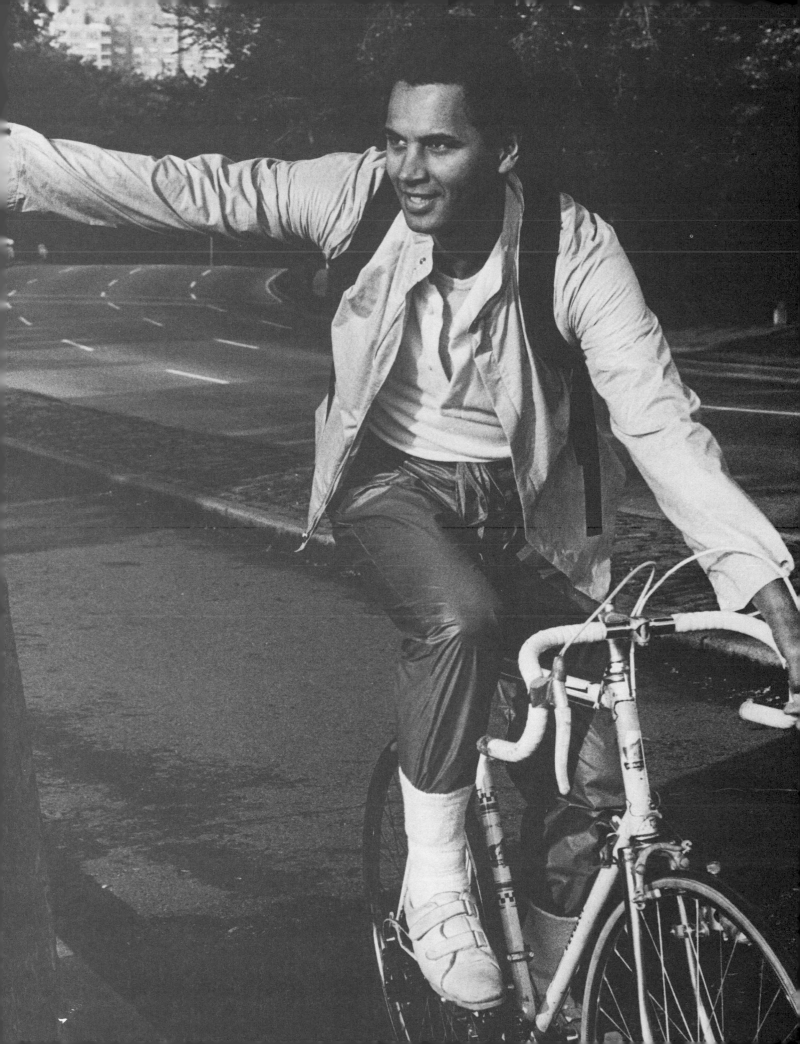

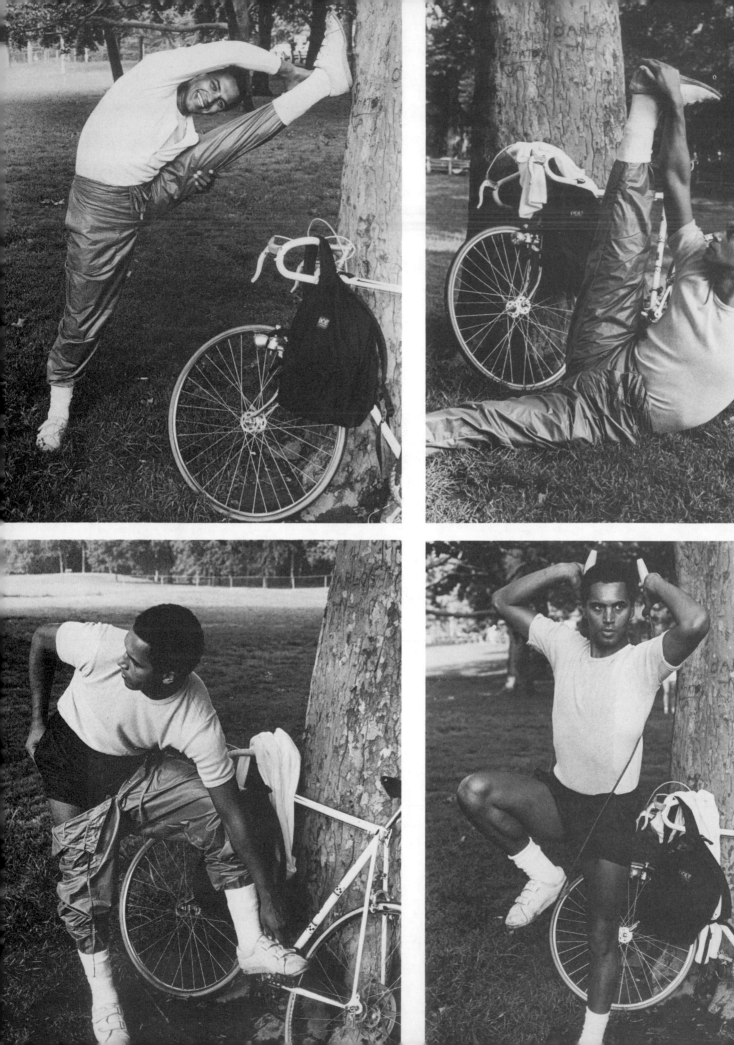

HOT STUFF

Clothing isn't warm. Your body is. A lumberjack plaid flannel shirt is no warmer in a bureau drawer than a tie-dyed tank top. In fact, tucked away, they're at exactly the same temperature: the equivalent of the air surrounding them—what's referred to as ambient temperature. Only when you put on one or the other does it feel warm or cool. That's because you're a warm-blooded animal, and *you* supply the heat to warm yourself. You also supply the perspiration to cool yourself. Whether you feel snug as a bug or raw to the bone depends upon several factors, ambient temperature being only one of them.

When you exercise indoors, you can usually control the temperature—and, to a limited extent, how much you perspire—by flicking the thermostat. Since your body generates progressively more heat during a workout, a cool environment—about 65 degrees Fahrenheit—is ideal.

Outdoors, the heat (or cold) is not adjustable. When exercising outside, you must adjust your activities—and/or your clothing—to the climate.

Cold weather presents less difficulty than sultry temperatures. Even frigid air is warmed before it reaches the lungs, so they're not going to freeze. If you dress protectively, there's little to fear if you keep attuned to body reactions.

In cold weather, your body conserves heat by slowing down circulation to the skin, thereby concentrating warmth internally. Although your extremities feel cooler, your body maintains its normal temperature. However, as you exercise, your blood heads out to the skin again, warming your extremities. Owing to the exercise, your internal temperature remains normal. Should you become so active that your insides heat up, you perspire to normalize your temperature once more even in an arctic setting.

Hot, humid weather is more problematical, because the body's temperature isn't much greater than the external temperature. Perspiration can't cool the body as it normally does because evaporation is slow when there's little or no inside/outside temperature differential. The body just keeps heating up, perspiration being insufficient to cool it, which can lead to exhaustion or heatstroke.

The only way to acclimate yourself to working out

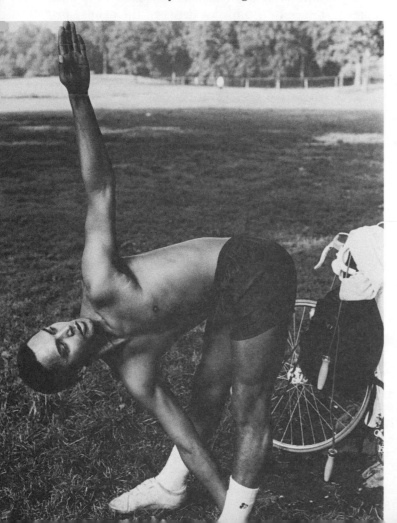
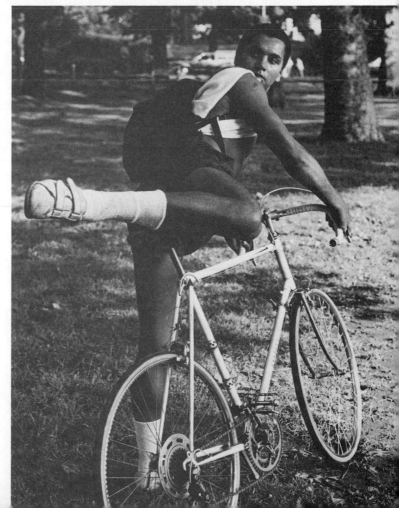

WARM-WEATHER EXERCISE

Radiant heat from the sun makes you feel hotter than you really are, and if your skin is unprotected, bright sun can produce a bright burn. For these reasons, it's better to wear something than nothing. (Exercising dressed also saves you legal fees.) But the something should not be thick, dark garb. White clothing deflects the sun's rays, while dark-colored attire absorbs them, making you hotter. However, fair warning: Wet white clothing sometimes lets through the rays, causing you to burn.

Mesh shirts are good for outdoor warm-weather exercise because they encourage perspiration evaporation. On the other hand, being porous, they don't keep out the sun as much as more tightly woven tops do.

Terry and velour absorb sweat, so initially they can feel more comfortable than less absorbent materials. However, once they're drenched they're no better than any other fabrics.

Hairy or fuzzy fabrics should be avoided for two reasons. One, with their numerous open spaces, they catch and hold hot air. Two, they are less soothing to the skin than flat-surfaced materials. Ironed exercise garb has more contact with your skin and feels better than wrinkled attire. Why? Unless the temperature is tropical, the air surrounding you is cooler than your body. Your exercise clothes will consequently be cooler in temperature too, nearly the same as the ambient reading. The more contact your skin makes with the cooler clothing, the more body heat you lose through conduction. Since smooth, ironed fabrics touch your skin more directly and completely than wrinkled or fuzzy ones, you just feel cooler wearing them although your internal temperature is about the same.

Because you want to minimize clothing's insulation during hot spells, you will gravitate toward thin fabrics that retain less air than thicker ones.

The hotter you get in hot and humid weather, the more difficult it is for you to stay even remotely cool. Tight bikini underwear, even a jock, makes you that much hotter. Although it's not a modest thing to do, you'll be more comfortable skipping undergarments entirely in favor of smooth gym shorts that feel good next to the skin. This is also a very revealing thing to do, and you could be accused of exhibitionism.

in high temperatures is purposefully to work yourself into a dripping sweat every time you exercise. But it's always harder to perform in torrid heat than in frigid cold, and clothing can be a trouble at both extremes.

Atop your body but beneath the vagaries of style, all clothing is basically insulation. First, every garment you put on traps air between the skin's surface and the article of clothing itself, unless the fabric is meshlike and allows air to escape. Second,

COLD-WEATHER EXERCISE

You require fewer layers of clothing to exercise in the cold than to sit on a park bench admiring a winterscape. As long as you remain physically active, your body generates more heat than usual. However, once you stop exercising, your body puts out less heat and you feel cold if you don't layer up.

Layering exercise garb is the only way to outsmart a plummeting mercury. Your first layer should be fairly thin and absorbent. The outer layer should *not* be very absorbent, because if it becomes wet, you lose more heat. (Water is a good conductor and draws body heat away from you, releasing it in the atmosphere.) Wool is a good top layer because it dries from the inside out (assuming it's not raining). With its outside relatively dry, wool provides good insulation for as long as you wear it even if the inside is dampened by perspiration.

Nonbreathing synthetic fibers are questionable top layers. They don't allow the wind to penetrate them—a point in their favor; but they also don't allow perspiration to get out—a demerit, since you can feel clammy after working up a sweat.

Down makes a good middle layer because of its thickness and lightness.

Of course, wearing several layers of clothing does reduce your mobility, making coordinated exercise more difficult. That's the main reason indoor exercise is preferable to outdoor activity when the weather's numbing: It's simply harder to work out well when encumbered with layers of clothes.

Meanwhile, while cheating the cold by working out indoors, think about practical considerations. Don't buy gym shorts with buckles or buttons; they will jab you while you're working out, especially during your limbering routine. An elasticized waistband is preferred, but not one so snug it chafes.

For tops, sleeveless are generally best, although they don't curb the flow of sweat spilling from your armpits. Sweat shirts are okay until they're too sweaty. Ultimately, going topless is a valid and viable alternative.

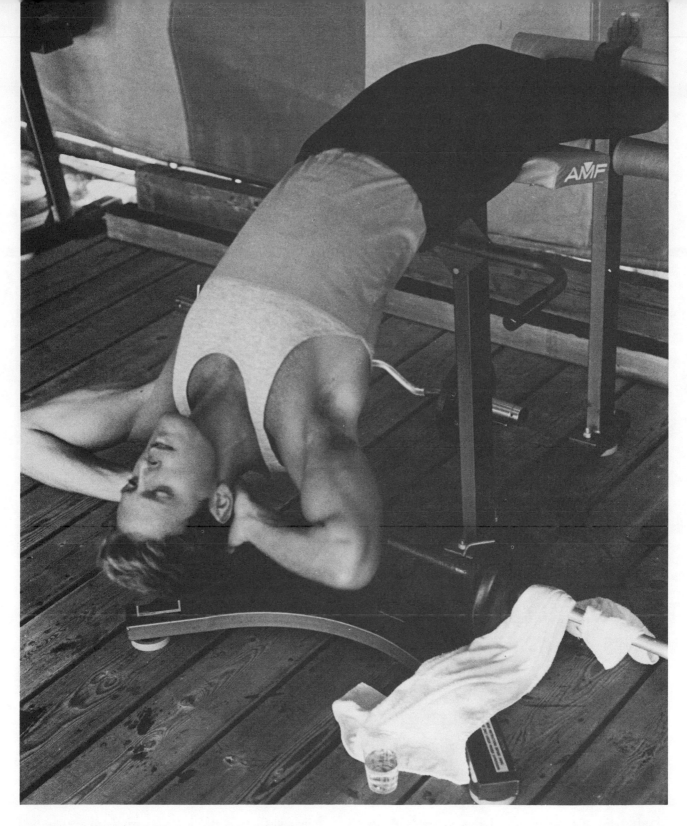

garments themselves hold air. Thick, nubbly textured fabrics retain more air than thin, slick ones. The more air a fabric contains, the warmer it feels because it is more insulating, valiantly resistant to liberating body heat from its tactile clutches. This is great in cold climes, not so terrific in hot spots.

When you wear several layers of clothing, you snare more air, supplementing insulation. Piling on three or four sweaters is more insulating, hence more warming, than swaddling yourself in a horse blanket.

Tight clothing makes it more difficult for air to escape than looser garments which allow air to circulate more freely. When air circulates, you lose

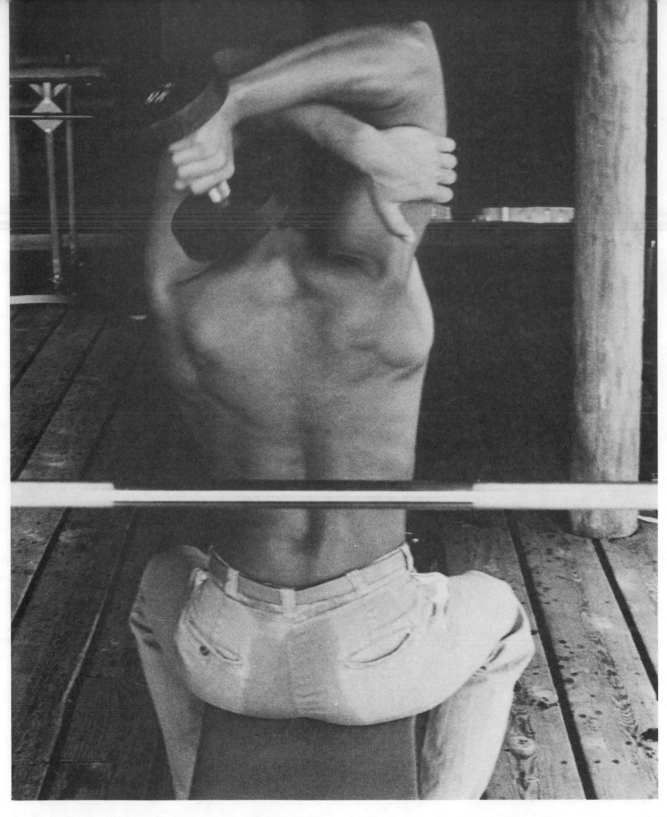

body heat. Consequently, when your aim is fighting the cold, you want to keep air from circulating, holding it next to your body or between clothing layers, which pretty much amounts to the same thing. (Down-filled vests are warmer than tight leather ones, for example, because the downy numbers are thicker with air pockets. Likewise, baggy pants elasticized at the ankles are warmer than tight jeans for a similar reason: The baggies entrap more air, which the elasticized ankles won't let out.)

Generally, when you're working out, you're more intent as the session progresses on heat loss than on heat retention or gain, because you're stoking up more energy through physical activity.

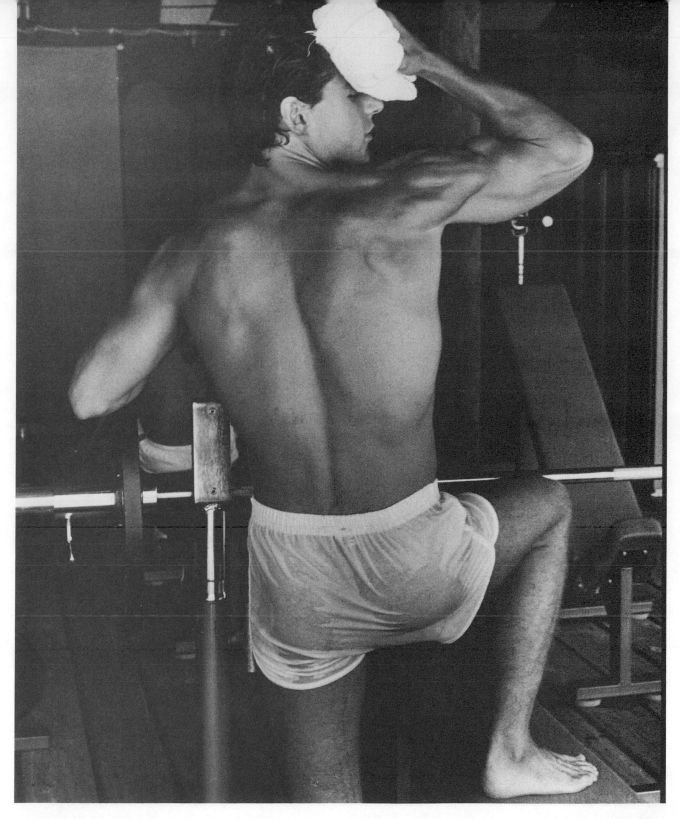

Loose exercise garb is always more air-circulating than tight attire—another reason to opt for looseness and comfort. Exercising in the nude is the coolest way, but you might feel a little odd. Particularly if you work out at a gym. Your membership might be revoked.

Indoors, if a fan is handy, you can always encourage heat loss by creating an artificial breeze. Outdoors, you must rely on your layering—or disrobing—ingenuity. Regardless, once you've worked out and shaped up, you—and your body—will look great whatever you wear. Or whatever you don't.

INDEX

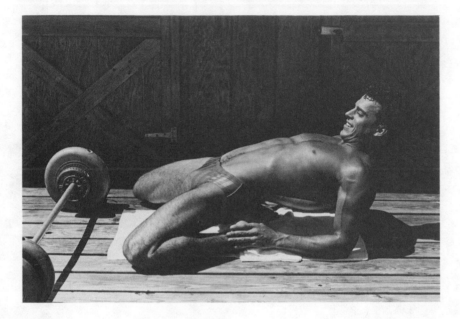

224